WHEAT BELLY

10-DAY DETOX

By the same author

Wheat Belly
Wheat Belly Cookbook
Wheat Belly 30-Minute (or Less!) Cookbook
Wheat Belly Total Health

DR WILLIAM DAVIS

WHEAT BELLY

10-DAY DETOX

**THE GRAIN-FREE PLAN TO REPROGRAMME
YOUR BODY FOR RAPID WEIGHT LOSS
AND AMAZING HEALTH**

Thorsons

Thorsons
An imprint of HarperCollins*Publishers*
1 London Bridge Street
London SE1 9GF

www.harpercollins.co.uk

First published in this edition by Rodale Inc. 2015
Published in Great Britain by Thorsons 2016

1 3 5 7 9 10 8 6 4 2

© William Davis 2015

Book design by Amy King

William Davis asserts the moral right to be
identified as the author of this work

A catalogue record of this book is
available from the British Library

ISBN 978-0-00-814677-1

This book is intended as a reference volume only, not as a medical manual.
The information given here is designed to help you make informed decisions
about your health. It is not intended as a substitute for any treatment that may
have been prescribed by your doctor. If you suspect that you have a medical
problem, we urge you to seek competent medical help. Mention of specific
companies, organisations or authorities in this book does not imply endorsement
by the author or publisher nor does mention of specific companies, organisations
or authorities imply that they endorse this book, its author or the publisher.
In order to protect the privacy of patients, some names and
personal details have been changed.

Internet addresses given in this book were accurate at the time it went to press.

Printed and bound in Great Britain by Clays Ltd, St Ives plc

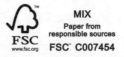

MIX
Paper from
responsible sources
FSC® C007454

FSC is a non-profit international organisation established to promote
the responsible management of the world's forests. Products carrying
the FSC label are independently certified to assure consumers that they
come from forests that are managed to meet the social, economic
and ecological needs of present and future generations.

Find out more about HarperCollins and the environment at
www.harpercollins.co.uk/green

To all the readers who have come to understand that health begins with personal effort, not with doctors, drugs, or the "health care" system.

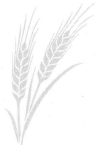

CONTENTS

ACKNOWLEDGMENTS

SINCE THE ORIGINAL *Wheat Belly* book was released in August 2011, the Wheat Belly movement has continued to grow. It is now an international phenomenon, with the book now published in 33 countries.

Despite that growth, I still regard the several million people following these concepts to be "early adopters," those people first in line who are brave enough to buck conventional dietary "wisdom" and who have come to recognize just how powerful this lifestyle can be in regaining control over health and weight. These bold individuals are the force that is expanding the reach of this message. It is time to take this message to the broader public, the same people who lament their size 28 dresses, 40-inch waists, and scales registering north of 200 pounds, and who are growing increasingly unhealthy and weighed down by the drugs used to "treat" a diet gone wrong—yet blame it on personal weakness or a bad draw of the genetic cards. This most recent addition to the Wheat Belly series is designed to make the process as digestible as possible.

The inspiration for this 10-day detox concept came from my team at Rodale, namely Editorial Director Jennifer Levesque, Deputy Publisher Kristin Kiser, and Publisher Mary Ann Naples. I therefore owe a big thank-you to all involved who helped make this detox project a mainstream-focused effort.

I also owe a big thank-you to Michele Stanten, author and vocal advocate of walking as exercise, who took time from her busy schedule to help organize the detox panelists' experiences chronicled in this book. Michele enlisted the panelists from the start, helped educate them on how to conduct this lifestyle, and supported them through the process. She played a crucial and indispensable role from start to finish. Thanks, Michele.

And thank you to the panelists, women who traveled to my American publisher's offices in New York from as far away as Texas and Georgia to participate in this detox process. Your participation helped make this program better, helped refine several of the recipes, and reminded me of the real challenges that readers face when they take this program into their homes and families.

My agent, Rick Broadhead, has been my advocate from the start of the Wheat Belly journey. Rick has been more than a literary agent: He has been objective observer, champion of the cause, and friend. As with every other book in the Wheat Belly series, I owe Rick another big thank-you.

I'd like to also acknowledge the countless individuals who have participated in online conversations on Wheat Belly social media, especially the Wheat Belly Facebook page, as they have engaged in this journey with me—all the people who have shared their wonderful "before" and "after" photos, their health successes, and their challenges, helping all of us learn new lessons that make this program more and more effective and less and less disruptive to daily routines. I am a big believer in the power of the wisdom of crowds, and this is, to a large degree, what we are creating with the Wheat Belly movement: a level of insight and wisdom that exceeds what any single expert could provide, but emerging with strategies for health and weight that are more powerful than anything ever conceived. It is a powerful force that I believe we have distilled and encapsulated in this book, the most recent addition to the Wheat Belly library. Thank you to all of you.

INTRODUCTION

WHAT IF I could provide you with a miraculous pill that caused dramatic weight loss without limiting calories or requiring exercise? What if this pill reduced appetite, shrunk belly fat, dropped your dress size into the single digits, and accomplished all this while sparing you from a *Biggest Loser* sobfest? What if that same pill freed you from acid reflux, heartburn, bowel urgency, and diarrhea, but also improved mood, increased energy, deepened sleep, and reduced or eliminated joint pain? What if this pill also reversed skin conditions such as seborrhea, eczema, psoriasis, acne, and dandruff and earned you compliments on the smoothness of your skin? What if chronic sinus congestion, sinus infections, and asthma were brought to a halt and you were freed from the repeated need for antibiotics and inhalers? What if that same little pill, taken every day, reversed serious inflammatory conditions such as rheumatoid arthritis, Crohn's disease, and ulcerative colitis, while causing your teenage children to put down their cell phones, be respectful, bathe without asking every day, and pick up their own clothes?

Okay, forget the part about teenagers. But what if this single pill could also replace cholesterol drugs, blood pressure drugs, diabetes drugs, anti-inflammatory drugs, antidepressants, and acid reflux drugs while reducing cholesterol values, blood sugars, and inflammation—packing the power of dozens of prescription medications into one pill but with none of the side effects? And what if this same powerful pill not only made you *feel* better than you have in years but also had the potential to achieve a physical makeover that made you *look* 10, even 20, years younger without

Botox, filler injections, or marriage to Kanye West, without unwanted health consequences but still the unmitigated envy at your 20-, 30-, or 40-year high school reunion?

And, unlike a fistful of daily pills costing hundreds of dollars every month, often adding up to more than your grocery bill, this one pill is inexpensive, even yielding cost savings—money you can put toward a new wardrobe.

Does such a miraculous pill exist that accomplishes this entire list of health and weight benefits at virtually no cost?

No, it does not. If someone told you it did, it would be a blatant instance of "too good to be true." There is certainly no such magical pill among the thousands of prescription drugs available. Prescription weight-loss drugs that yield billions of dollars per year for the drug industry come with a long list of potential side effects, from diarrhea to damaged heart valves, not to mention the return of the weight when you stop taking the drugs. Anti-inflammatory drugs commonly cause bleeding stomach ulcers, fluid retention, hypertension, and weight gain. Cholesterol-reducing drugs increase risk for diabetes, impair memory, and can cause muscle aches and weakness, making it difficult to even get in or out of a car. Drugs for erectile dysfunction can cause blindness, and in my view an unjustifiable dent in the wallet, and bad TV commercials.

A perfect drug to achieve even one of the benefits listed—let alone the entire list—simply does not exist, despite the extraordinary sums spent to promote them. Likewise, nutritional supplements: As much as I adore nutritional supplements for their power to achieve goals in health, there is no single supplement (nor list of supplements) that can achieve this entire list of benefits. Not even close.

But it does exist, not as a pill, but as a change in lifestyle, a simple collection of health strategies that can achieve all the benefits in the above list. Too good to be true? Hardly.

By far the most powerful factor in this lifestyle that gets the entire process started is to eliminate all foods made of wheat and grains—yes, the foods you were told to eat more of, told should dominate all meals from breakfast and lunch to dinner and snacks. The foods you were told to consume many times per day every day, the widest part of the food pyramid, the largest slice of the food plate, the darling of all conventional dietary advice and agribusiness. These are the foods that most weigh you down and ravage your health, worse than the "friend" who booby-traps your every move.

The worst dietary advice ever conceived tells you to reduce fat, eat more "healthy whole grains," and eat everything in moderation. Following this advice does not make you thinner and does not reverse health conditions, but only causes them or makes them worse. Removing wheat and grains from your life yields such outsized and unexpected health and weight benefits that it seems impossible, until you witness it day after day and experience it yourself.

The Wheat Belly 10-Day Detox is unlike all other detox programs. It does not involve cleansing your body with various juices or a magical concoction of supplements purported to remove body "toxins," nor is it a timetable of daily enemas that complicate your meeting schedule. It is a detoxification process from the toxic effects of wheat and grains, a detoxification in the truest sense of the term. But it is not just a matter of *not* eating wheat and grains or of eating "gluten-free" (as critics often perceive it). Once the toxic effects of wheat and grains have been removed, additional steps are necessary to undo the entire range of ill effects accumulated from their consumption.

This 10-day detox distills all the wisdom of the original Wheat Belly books and the lessons learned by the millions of people who have adopted this approach—incorporating the most insightful, cutting-edge, and effective strategies, and sharing them with you so that you can begin your path to weight and health success in a short 10 days. This lightning-fast approach has never been detailed in any previous Wheat Belly book.

I start with an overview of the program, give you specific how-tos on shopping and restocking your kitchen, and provide a detailed 10-Day Menu Plan. I also provide you with additional recipes to create little snack morsels that can be used to subdue cravings that crop up during your detox, as well as "Secret Weapon" recipes to help deal with family misgivings. I will also discuss the nutritional supplements we add to take your health even higher and help you feel even better—probably the best you've felt in a good long time. I will also share many of the comments and experiences provided by a courageous group of Wheat Belly 10-Day Detox panelists who blazed the path for you and engaged in the detox to help illustrate what you can expect. They will tell you why they engaged in this program, what they felt along the way, and the results they experienced even within these 10 days. While they reported some pretty impressive results, I believe they will tell you that the process was not all fun and games, but serious results require some serious methods!

You are going to learn that the grain detoxification process begins with enduring a genuine withdrawal syndrome similar to that experienced with stopping any narcotic. We will discuss this in some detail so that you don't misinterpret its meaning and tell yourself that you must need wheat and grains to avoid such unpleasant effects. I will also discuss how we can smooth over (though not entirely eliminate) the withdrawal process, making it less difficult to endure. The first few days of the grain detoxification process are therefore crucial. Only after getting this process behind you will it be possible to take steps to reverse the organ damage incurred and begin the process of healing.

The science and rationale behind this powerful approach was discussed at length in the original book, *Wheat Belly*, and its follow-up, *Wheat Belly Total Health*. This book, *Wheat Belly 10-Day*

Detox, is designed for both newcomers as well as those of you who have strayed from the Wheat Belly lifestyle but wish to make a comeback. If you are among those who strayed—and you reacquired all the health and weight problems that come with resuming wheat and grain consumption—this book will get you back on track as fast and efficiently as possible without bogging you down with another discussion of the science and rationale.

The 10-Day Menu Plan, never before used in any other Wheat Belly book, provides a detailed day-by-day road map to keep you on course—or get you back on course—with plenty of delicious, easy-to-prepare recipes. They are all consistent with the Wheat Belly lifestyle and tasty enough to be served to your family, whether or not they are engaging in this lifestyle with you.

This hard-hitting how-to has only the most essential tools required to get you started and take you from zero to 60 miles per hour and on the road back to slenderness and health with breathtaking speed. Though I'm leaving out most of the science that validates this approach, suffice it to say that wheat and grains impair health in so many ways that most people never even suspect that the high-fiber cereal in their breakfast bowl every morning created the "muffin top" they're trying to conceal under baggy tops and multilayered one-piece bathing suits, as well as their knee pain, migraines, and asthma. Most people never suspect that the annoying, itchy, embarrassing rash they've endured for the past 10 years; the crippling joint pain in their hands that complicates the simplest tasks like brushing teeth or writing a check; the need to run to the toilet for an uninvited loose bowel movement; or the constant struggle with constipation, anxiety, depression, headaches, and sinus congestion can all be due to "healthy whole grain" bread, bran muffins, or licorice (yes, licorice is a grain-containing food). People are shocked to learn that fatty liver and high blood sugars, the infertility of polycystic ovarian syndrome, and the embarrassment of man breasts and erectile dysfunction are not due to moral weakness, lack of discipline, or lack of access to better health care, but are grain induced.

Grains have posed a host of health problems for as long as humans have consumed them. But it became much more obvious when agribusiness genetically altered the favorite of all conventional "healthy foods," wheat, creating modern 18-inch-tall semi-dwarf strains for increased yield that replaced the 5-foot-tall "amber waves of grain" we all remember. Its destructive health effects were compounded by conventional dietary advice to eat more of it, while food manufacturers put wheat, corn, and other grains into virtually every processed food on store shelves, taking the "eat more healthy whole grains" message to an absurd extreme.

One of the reasons why it was so difficult for people to draw cause-effect relationships between wheat and grains and this long list of health problems is that most of the effects are delayed and only show themselves over the long term. A stack of waffles eaten on May 1 may not yield, for instance, the swollen joints and pain of rheumatoid arthritis until September 30 or later, so it's tough to connect the dots. But the dots do indeed connect.

So the Wheat Belly 10-Day Detox is not only the nutritional equivalent of a magical pill that can achieve all the above benefits, but also a rejection of the "eat more healthy whole grains" and other dietary advice we hear repeated over and over again. We are going to thumb our noses at the food pyramid and plate, turn a deaf ear to the advice of organizations like the American Diabetes and American Heart Associations, and snicker at the marketing antics of Big Food eager to sell us their cellophane-wrapped, processed foods packed with grains and sugar—all while you get closer and closer to fitting into size 8 jeans, pitching most, if not all, of your prescription drugs into the trash, and feeling the best you have in decades.

Yes, many of the prescription drugs that your doctor advised you to take are really efforts to treat the consequences of eating a diet centered on "healthy whole grains" and the grain-tainted products that fill processed supermarket foods. Being released from these effects does not involve cutting calories, reducing fat, prolonged periods of denial, restraint, or exercise. Get rid of the cause, reverse the effect: The start of this process is really that simple.

Ten days—a week and a half, a third of a month, the time it takes to order and receive a new pair of shoes online—and you can chart a new course for your life and enjoy the wonderful benefits of reprogramming your body along an entirely new design. Once you have gotten through the next 10 days and emerge thinner, faster, stronger, smarter, and healthier for less than the cost of a pair of new shoes, you will wonder what you were thinking over the preceding 30, 40, or 50 years. Your health and your appearance are likely to draw gasps from anyone who witnesses the "after" who lived with your "before."

So let's begin!

CHAPTER 1

YOU'VE BEEN ROLLED, TOSSED, AND BAKED

"Follow a balanced diet low in fat."

"You need whole grains for B vitamins and fiber."

"It's unhealthy to eliminate an entire food group."

"Everything in moderation."

THIS SHOULD ALL sound familiar to you because these nutritional mantras have been repeated over and over by dietitians, doctors, and the media. And, like many such pieces of conventional "wisdom," there is a germ of truth in each of them—but just a germ and nothing more. Following such advice not only does *not* help you control weight or obtain health, it also destroys your grasp over weight and health. It can be as ineffective as believing that total health is restored by taking a prescription drug, subjecting yourself to a 4-week program of "cleansing" enemas, or concealing bulges under a new set of Spanx. Modern misguided dietary advice has made plus-size aisles the busiest place in clothing stores, huffing and puffing commonplace when climbing a single flight of stairs, and type 2 diabetes a double-digit growth industry.

Don't feel bad if you fell for it, choosing lean cuts and trimming the fat off meat, reaching for low-fat yogurt, and opting for whole grain breads, muffins, and bagels. Many beliefs, once accepted as gospel, have fallen by the wayside over the years, kicked to the curb by new discoveries, new science, and new understanding. It wasn't all that long ago that you would have been burned at the stake for believing that the earth revolved around the sun, been prosecuted for voicing the wrong political views during the McCarthy-era purges, or cheered for Milli Vanilli's "Girl You Know It's True" win at the Grammy Awards. Human history is filled with such campaigns of misinformation. But only in the recent past has misinformation permeated nutritional advice on such a grand scale.

HALF-BAKED

When you lose control over your health and weight because you ate "healthy" whole grains, doctors—stumped by why you feel so awful despite doing everything "right"—prescribe drugs with effects that create the "need" for even more prescription drugs. This is the modern downward health spiral that most people find themselves trapped in today. Once you understand this absurd and self-defeating situation, you are empowered to change it. And you can begin to powerfully reverse this situation over the next 10 days, the number of days it takes your husband to stop procrastinating over fixing a leaky kitchen faucet. This detox process yields a head-to-toe body and health makeover, reprogramming your body at so many levels, both internal and external. Your body and health will undergo a transformation that may even have friends and family not believing it's you.

With the bad science and politics that drove the "cut your cholesterol, fat, and saturated fat" agenda of the latter half of the 20th century, the bonfire was lit even brighter by over-the-top profit opportunities for Big Food. The low-fat message gained a huge following. In its wake now lies the result: obesity, diabetes, arthritis, dementia, and other health disasters on a scale never before witnessed in the history of mankind. It's an unprecedented

man-made social and health apocalypse that makes reports of tor-
nadoes and radiation spills seem like small-scale annoyances, even
banal, with nearly two billion overweight or obese people worldwide (including nearly 50 million children under age 5) and more
than half of Americans with diabetes or prediabetes. The low-fat
message, because it eliminated a source of satiating calories from
fat, caused everyone to resort to more carbohydrates, particularly
the carbohydrate source that most nutritional authorities felt to
be the healthiest: whole grains, such as whole wheat, oats, and rye.

But, like the message to cut fat and saturated fat—now
debunked by more recent studies showing that fat and saturated
fat have nothing to do with cardiovascular disease—so the "eat
more healthy whole grains" message was also based on flawed science and misinterpretations. The purported health benefits of
whole grains were based on epidemiological studies (i.e., studies
of health in large populations) demonstrating that if white flour
products are replaced with whole grains, there is less diabetes, less
weight gain, less heart disease, and less colon cancer in the population observed. That is indeed true and not in question. Careers
and entire university departments of nutrition have been built on
this premise. But the next question should have been: What is the
effect of removing grains, white and whole, altogether? We cannot answer that question with the same "replace one with the
other" epidemiological studies; we have to look elsewhere. Such
grain-eliminating studies have indeed already been performed.

What happens when we remove grains? Clinical studies have
shown:

- Weight loss (not less weight gain)
- Reduction in overall calorie intake
- Drops in blood sugar and hemoglobin A1c (a long-term mea-
  sure of blood sugar)—many people with diabetes are cured
- Reduction of blood pressure
- Increased likelihood of remission of rheumatoid arthritis

- Reversal of neurological conditions such as cerebellar ataxia, some forms of seizures, and peripheral neuropathy
- Reversal of multiple forms of skin rash
- Reductions in paranoia and hallucinations in people with schizophrenia
- Improved attention span and behavior in children with attention deficit disorder and autistic spectrum disorder
- Relief from the bowel urgency and disruption of irritable bowel syndrome

That's just a sample of the evidence that already exists in the scientific and clinical literature. This is not conjecture or claims based on a few anecdotes. It is based on a rational, scientific examination of the evidence, coupled with the experiences of millions of people who have come to understand the power of this lifestyle change. When a wheat- and grain-free lifestyle is put to work in real life, the benefits documented in clinical studies can be seen in action with unexpected and dramatic reversal of numerous health conditions.

Such a collection of changes is rare to impossible when weight loss is achieved through a painful few weeks of calorie counting, liposuction, or kickboxing or other strenuous exercise. If this were just a weight-loss program or just a program to shrink your waist, well, that would be sort of interesting in a reality TV sort of way, complete with emotional outbursts and breakdowns. But it would not be accompanied by the sorts of body and health transformations we are seeking. In this detoxification process, we are going to go further than just losing weight; we are going to work to restore health from head to toe. Weight loss, feeling better, and looking younger are simply reflections of the dramatic improvements in health you are going to experience.

In particular, you are likely to experience a powerful reversal of inflammation throughout your body. The reversal of redness, swelling, pain, and hormonal signal disruption that we may experience variously as seborrhea, rheumatoid arthritis, acid reflux, leg swelling, or irrational anger all reflect the receding wave of inflammation previously caused by grains.

These are changes that I observe in people every day with the health strategies detailed in the Wheat Belly books. In this easy-to-consume, bite-size book, you will read about such changes from our detox panelists, even in the brief 10-day timeline of this program. I predict that many of you, like our volunteer panelists, will receive compliments from family and friends after these initial 10 days on how different you look: thinner, yes, but it's not uncommon for your appearance to begin to change, especially that of the face with less eye puffiness, less facial edema, and relief from the redness of the cheeks and seborrhea along the nose (what I call the signature rashes of wheat and related grains), as well as developing better defined facial contours, reduced waist size, smaller hips, reduced cellulite on the thighs, loss of edema in the ankles, even smaller feet—no kidding. I bet you'll even smile more readily, given how much better you feel inside.

The Wheat Belly 10-Day Detox program begins with the elimination of wheat and grains, the essential first step that gets the detoxification process under way. But this detox involves additional strategies for full benefit. These strategies are necessary because they undo many of the unhealthy effects that grains have exerted on your body and that have accumulated over the years, such as abnormal rises in insulin levels and altered composition of bowel flora (the microorganisms that inhabit your intestinal tract). Many of the drugs that your doctor prescribed to treat the destructive health effects of wheat and grain consumption will also need to be reduced or discarded. Remove the initial cause, correct the varied consequences, and the majority of drugs are no longer needed and health can finally reassert itself. Without grains, life is indeed good.

These sorts of benefits have nothing to do with celiac disease, the autoimmune destruction of the small intestine from gluten in wheat, rye, and barley experienced by 1 percent of the population. While this detox program could be undertaken by someone with celiac disease, it is primarily aimed at people without the disease, meaning the other 99 percent of the population. These ben-

Wheat Belly 10-Day Detox Put to the Test

In March 2015, my American publisher and I invited a group of volunteers to Rodale's Manhattan offices to undergo an initiation to the Wheat Belly 10-Day Detox program. I had posted a request for volunteers on the Wheat Belly Facebook page and received an outpouring of offers to participate. All panelists shared an interest in getting started on the detox program and obtaining results as quickly as possible. While most expressed a desire to lose weight, all hoped to regain control over various health conditions.

The panelists (all female) in our group came from different parts of the country. To get them started on this process, we helped them understand a bit about why this lifestyle works so wonderfully well, but just as with the rapid-fire approach used in this book, we focused mostly on the *how:* how to identify grain-containing foods, how to go about eliminating them from their lives, and how to successfully navigate the first 10 days of the detox, including how to deal with the uncomfortable and disruptive process of withdrawal to begin a lifetime of health recovery.

We provided them with the very same recipes that you now have in this book, asking them for feedback, which was then factored in, and we improved on some of the recipes. We weighed them and measured their waists, arms, and hips on the first and last days of the detox. We also asked them for their thoughts on how they dealt with this process; the symptoms, aches, and pains they endured; and any health improvements they experienced. They shared their successes, their failures, the ups and downs of the process, the struggles with converting their kitchens to this new wheat- and grain-free lifestyle, and the sometimes reluctant or skeptical looks they got from family members.

I will be sharing many of the panelists' experiences throughout this book. They all underwent the very same detox program that you are about to begin. All survived and lived to tell their stories.

efits also have little to do with being "gluten-free," a misleading concept that has the potential to ruin health and weight in other ways, which we'll discuss throughout the book.

You will learn also that not only will you not become deficient in nutrients, but that nutrient levels *increase* with wheat and grain elimination—explaining why, for example, many people experience reversal of iron deficiency anemia and vitamin B_{12} deficiency with this approach. I also take the mystery out of fiber and show why the conventional notion of a high-fiber diet is largely a fiction of marketing, little different than sprinkling sawdust on your food. There are better ways to achieve bowel and overall health than gnawing on twigs.

The Wheat Belly 10-Day Detox therefore requires not only changes in lifestyle but also changes in your thinking about food and nutrition. Replacing your size 24, meant-to-conceal dress with a sleek, size 8 dress designed to show off your slender new body will go hand in hand with changes in the way you view food, replacing the health- and weight-destroying fictions with advice that actually works.

GRAINS: A HEALTH AND WEIGHT CATASTROPHE

I promised to spare you the science and rationale behind the Wheat Belly concepts. But allow me to sprinkle just a bit of understanding over why this approach works so wonderfully well—so much so that I am sometimes accused of concocting success stories. But I can assure you that no fabrication is necessary because (1) I really don't have that much imagination, and (2) such jaw-dropping successes occur every day, and we can readily add you to the list. I believe that just a little explanation is in order to assure you that this approach is genuine, based on scientific interpretation, not only anecdote or speculation, and that real results can be anticipated.

I call wheat and grain elimination a "2 + 2 = 11" effect: The total in this lifestyle is greater than the sum of its parts. Some people initially view the Wheat Belly approach as nothing more than cutting calories or cutting carbohydrates. But this is a misconception due to not recognizing all the reasons why wheat and grains disrupt health and why removing them yields larger-than-expected benefits. Removing all the factors in grains responsible for inflammation, for instance, results in a wide array of weight and health benefits.

So let's do a quick rundown of what is contained in the wheat and grains that make a bran muffin, poppy seed bagel, or tortilla poisonous components of diet. I'll keep it brief, and then we'll pick up again with workable strategies to get you going.

GRAINS YIELD OPIATES. Not figuratively, but quite literally, these opiates are not too different from morphine or heroin. Chances are you are not a pill-popping, tourniquet-on-the-bicep, IV drug–injecting, fringe member of society slinking in corners and dealing in the dark, but rather a nice, law-abiding member of society. The gliadin protein of wheat and closely related proteins of other grains (secalin in rye, hordein in barley, zein in corn) yield, upon partial digestion, small peptides that bind to the opiate receptors of the human brain. In people with conditions such as bipolar illness and schizophrenia, they yield effects such as impulsive behavior and paranoia; in children with attention deficit disorder and autism, they cause behavioral outbursts and shorten attention spans; in people prone to bulimia and binge eating disorder, they cause 24-hour-a-day food obsessions. In those prone to depression, they cause dark moods and even suicidal thoughts.

In people without these conditions, grains "only" trigger appetite in an irresistible, never-satisfied way. (Several of our detox panelists shared their experiences, by the way, of being relieved of this appetite effect that had previously ruled their lives.) Most of us take in 400 or more calories per day from this appetite-increasing effect, sometimes as much as 1,000 or more calories per day. Some people even develop incapacitating and addictive relationships with food due to exposure to gliadin-derived opiates, witnessed in their most extreme form as the food obsessions in people prone to eating disorders.

Yes, wheat and grains, cleverly disguised as a multigrain loaf of bread to make sandwiches or a hot, steamy plate of macaroni and cheese for the kids, are mind-active drugs. Your kids are not oxycodone addicts, but they eat wheat and grains; not all that different.

Stopping wheat and grains thereby yields an opiate-withdrawal syndrome (discussed in greater detail in Chapter 2), as well as a marked reduction in appetite. While you're in the Wheat Belly 10-Day Detox, I do *not* encourage calorie counting or cutting calories; however, if you were to tabulate calories, you would witness a substantial reduction in intake. (The reduction in calorie intake, by the way, is the basis for the Wheat Belly lifestyle usually not costing more money, despite our choice of higher-quality foods. If a family of five, for instance, experiences a reduction in calorie intake of 400 calories per person per day, that yields 2,000 fewer calories to purchase and prepare every day, 60,000 fewer calories per month. It's almost like not having to feed one person.) We will discuss why, during your first week when the detoxification/withdrawal process gets under way, you may not be the nicest person to be around (something our volunteers experienced firsthand and will share). We will also discuss how you can soften the blow of this effect and perhaps spare yourself from having to make embarrassed apologies to everyone around you at the end.

GRAINS INITIATE INFLAMMATION AND AUTOIMMUNITY. Many people with autoimmune conditions, such as rheumatoid arthritis, lupus, multiple sclerosis, Hashimoto's thyroiditis, seborrhea, psoriasis, or one of the other 200 such diseases, regard themselves as unlucky, having been dealt a faulty genetic hand that increases susceptibility to such serious conditions. There is some truth to that belief, but it is important to recognize that we now know that the gliadin protein of wheat, the secalin of rye, the hordein of barley, and the zein protein of corn initiate a series of steps in the human intestine that increase permeability, what some call gut leak. This allows the entry of foreign substances into the bloodstream, such as lipopolysaccharide from bacteria (a highly inflammatory molecule) and the gliadin protein molecule itself.

Gliadin is peculiar in that its structure resembles several human proteins, such as the transglutaminase enzyme in muscle or the synapsin protein in the brain, a peculiarity that allows it to do double duty: initiate intestinal leak, then provoke inflammation. Because of such similarities to human proteins, gliadin's presence in the human body causes a misdirected immune response against, for example, the cells of the brain containing synapsin, leading to degeneration of the cerebellum and resulting in progressive loss of balance and bladder control (cerebellar ataxia), or transglutaminase in the liver, causing the liver damage of autoimmune hepatitis. Different organs are targeted in different individuals, but much of it begins with the same phenomenon: abnormal intestinal permeability and inflammation from the components of grains passing through the intestines.

WHEAT GERM AGGLUTININ DISRUPTS DIGESTION. Wheat germ agglutinin, or WGA (contained in wheat, rye, barley, and rice), is a potent bowel toxin that is entirely resistant to human digestion. WGA blocks release of bile from the gallbladder and release of pancreatic enzymes from the pancreas, resulting in bile stasis and impaired digestion of food. This results in effects such as bowel urgency, incomplete food digestion, changes in bowel flora, and gallstones. WGA is also directly toxic to the gastrointestinal lining in its journey from mouth to toilet and highly inflammatory even in the small quantities that gain access into the bloodstream. WGA shares some structural similarities to ricin, a potent toxin used in terrorist attacks, only it doesn't come to you and your family through dirty bombs or contaminated water, but from a hot dog bun or a wrap.

AMYLOPECTIN A RAISES BLOOD SUGAR TO HIGH LEVELS. Even though we've been told that grains contain a "complex" carbohydrate, the unique branching structure of the carbohydrate in grains called amylopectin A makes it highly digestible by the enzyme amylase in saliva and the stomach, causing it to raise blood sugar, ounce for ounce, higher than table sugar. High blood sugars provoke high blood insulin; high blood insulin results in storing fat in fat cells, leading to weight gain. To make matters worse, after we consume grains, the resulting high blood sugars are followed by low blood sugars 90 to 120 minutes later, an effect accompanied by mental fogginess, fatigue, food cravings, and irrational lashing out at colleagues at work or school. Grain consumption therefore yields hunger in an uncomfortable and predictable 2-hour cycle, as well as a need for occasional requests for forgiveness.

PHYTATES BLOCK NUTRIENT ABSORPTION. Grains are full of phytates, compounds that block absorption of iron, zinc, magnesium, and other nutrients. (This is part of the reason why grains, such as breads, are fortified: to compensate for the nutrient-blocking effects of phytates.) Such deficiencies have implications of their own, including fatigue (if iron deficiency anemia develops), skin rashes and impaired immunity (from zinc deficiency), muscle cramps, disrupted blood sugar control, and bone thinning (from magnesium deficiency). Wheat and grain consumption is the second most common worldwide cause for iron deficiency anemia after blood loss. Given their phytate content, grains are about as nutritious as identity theft is good for your credit score. Grains are anti-nutrients.

That's a partial list of the components of grains that mess with health; there are more. With the exception of the highly digestible carbohydrate in grains, amylopectin A, you can detect a recurring theme in the problematic proteins of wheat and grains: They are indigestible or, at best, only partially digestible, unlike, say, the fully digestible proteins of an egg or piece of fish. If we recognize that grains—literally the seeds of grasses—were added to the human diet relatively recently in human history and added during a period of desperation (after all, who would intuitively or naturally view grasses as a source of calories?), it means that humans have had insufficient time to adapt. The indigestible or partially digestible proteins harvested from the seeds of grasses therefore exert peculiar effects on us, from mind effects to autoimmunity.

Such toxins come packaged in varied and delightful, enticing ways, such as cupcakes and kids' breakfast cereals, all gussied up

---

NICOLE, 48, flight attendant, Georgia

"If I had to pinpoint the motivation behind my grain-free journey, it would be the night my son ended up in the emergency room at midnight doubled over in pain with a severe stomachache. He had stomachaches before. Not on a daily basis, but periodically he would say his stomach hurt. Sometimes, he would feel like he had to vomit, other times he would sit on the toilet for what seemed like an hour. A lot of times he would miss school. A straight A student and gifted athlete. He had every reason to be angry and frustrated, and to have an 'I don't give a dang' attitude.

"I decided that night in the hospital, when they sent my son home with a painkiller and laxatives, that I was going to try to figure out what was wrong with him. I had him undergo allergy testing, which yielded no allergies. He was tested for celiac, Crohn's, and gluten intolerance. Nothing. I started documenting his food intake. I started noticing that he ate a lot of processed foods and easy-to-make things like sandwiches, pasta, and microwaved food. He was eating a LOT of grains. I found Dr. Davis on Facebook and immediately bought the first *Wheat Belly* book. After reading it, there was no doubt in my mind that my son was intolerant to grains.

"Little by little, I changed his diet. No more processed foods, no more pasta. His stomachaches started getting more infrequent, and there was a definite correlation between eating grains and his stomachaches. Sometimes the timing would be unusual, in that he would get a stomachache several days later after eating, say, chocolate chip cookies. But I could definitely see a connection."

with clever marketing, leading me to call wheat and grains perfect chronic poisons. I promised not to go into these effects any further, since my intention with the *Wheat Belly 10-Day Detox* is to help you get on track as fast as possible without getting bogged down in the science and rationale (those are discussed in the original *Wheat Belly: Lose the Wheat, Lose the Weight, and Find Your Path Back to Health* and in *Wheat Belly Total Health: The Ultimate Grain-Free Health and Weight-Loss Life Plan*). Rest assured that this book is not based on conjecture or anecdote; it is based on real science, solid rationale, and real results. But it is important to understand that the approach outlined here achieves such huge and unexpected results not because we are just cutting back calories or because we have only reduced carbohydrate intake. It works because we are eliminating the dozens of toxic compounds that live in wheat and grains.

FEED THE INSATIABLE MONSTER

You now know that there is a soup of toxic compounds in wheat and grains. This is true even if they are organic, traditional or heirloom, sprouted, or topped with your extra-special gravy. This is because grains contain such toxic components naturally, only made worse by recent genetic manipulations.

The amping up of appetite by wheat and grains, in particular, is worth discussing further for a moment. Gliadin-derived opiates drive appetite in an "I can never get enough to eat" way, as discussed above. The amylopectin A carbohydrate drives blood sugar highs, followed by blood sugar lows that launch a 2-hour cycle of hunger. But there's more.

WGA is also suspected of blocking leptin, the hormone of satiety charged with signaling your brain with a "stop eating" message when your stomach is full after, say, two trips to the all-you-can-eat buffet. In the presence of WGA, this signaling system is blocked, causing you to eat even after you are full, after you have taken in what you require for sustenance, making the chocolate cake, peach pie, and cheesecake at the end of the buffet irresistible—even when common sense, good judgment, and every other body signal tell you that you've had enough.

Making matters worse, high blood insulin provoked by amylopectin A causes belly fat to grow, viewed on the surface as a "muffin top" or "love handles" and seen on imaging tests such as CT scans as deep visceral fat encircling the abdominal organs. This belly fat is inflammatory fat that drives insulin levels up even further. Insulin causes fat storage and prevents mobilization of fat for energy. Eat grains, increase appetite, provoke high insulin, grow belly fat, increase inflammation, provoke even higher blood insulin—around and around it goes, a vicious cycle that ensures weight gain, the entire process initiated by a friendly looking blueberry muffin or bowl of organic oatmeal.

You'll find these phenomena reflected in the comments of some of our detox panelists, such as Rebecca, Alexandria, and Joan. All of them struggled mightily with incessant, unstoppable, insatiable appetites while eating grains, and all were magnificently relieved of this monster by banishing them.

This is why I call wheat and its closely related grains not just perfect chronic poisons, but also perfect obesogens: foods that are

---

YVETTE, 50, history professor, New Jersey

"The weight gain was really depressing. I had always been slender. Suddenly, I was a different person. Nothing in my wardrobe fit; my body felt like a stranger to me. I could tell that people were looking at me and wondering what happened. It's been humiliating and embarrassing. I just didn't feel like I had the mental energy to tackle a traditional diet such as Weight Watchers. A big part of our social life is sharing meals with our friends, and I like to cook and bake, and I did not want to give that up either. What I really want more than anything is just to get back to a place where I feel comfortable and healthy and confident in my own skin again."

perfectly crafted to make you fat, especially in the abdomen, what I call a wheat belly. If you have struggled to lose weight despite doing everything "right" while including plenty of "healthy whole grains," you now understand that you were actually following a weight *gain* program—not too different from a cigarette smoking cessation program that bases its success on smoking more cigarettes. If your waist size expanded, the scale registering higher and higher, while metabolic distortions like high blood sugar and triglycerides accumulated as you blamed yourself for weakness, gluttony, or sloth, well, you succeeded in allowing the perfect obesogens in wheat and grains to do their dirty work.

Understand these simple truths and you will understand why removing wheat and grains completely—without hesitation, without compromise, without a tearful goodbye—finally points you in the right direction, allowing control over weight and health. You were not weak, gluttonous, or slothful; you were feeding the insatiable monster created by eating grains.

We will also discuss why, once you are wheat- and grain-free, it is important to remain that way, or else you can be reexposed to their appetite- and weight-increasing effects. While one cookie or pretzel does not, of course, trigger a 30-pound weight gain by itself, all it takes is just one such indulgence and—bam!—the appetite-igniting effects return in all their lip-smacking, mind-clouding, bowel-agitating glory. I called this the "I ate one cookie and gained 30 pounds" effect in the original *Wheat Belly* book because I've seen it happen many times. Go wheat- and grain-free for, say, 3 months, then have a cookie or inadvertently get exposed to the flour in a sauce or bread crumbs in meat loaf, and your appetite is powerfully triggered, your resolve disintegrates, and your size 10 pants no longer fit. You regain 10, 20, or 30 pounds over a month because you lost control due to reexposure to all the components of grains. You may suffer some depression, mind "fog," joint pain, and diarrhea on top of it, as well. Some indulgence!

ELIZABETH, 48, sales consultant, New York

"I spent most of my adult life overweight. I exercised regularly and was probably cardiovascularly fit, but I was also anywhere from 40 to 80 pounds overweight. Then in 2010, I got breast cancer at 42. It was like a punch in the gut. I didn't see it coming. I was very fortunate that my cancer was treatable, and I had surgery to remove my left breast, then I started chemo about 6 weeks later. Chemo was awful. I have no words to describe how horrible it makes you feel. And one of the presents that I was left with after treatment was this chronic joint and muscle pain, mostly in my knees and legs, but also in my hips and upper back.

"I started reading up on grain elimination diets, and the part about wheat consumption triggering autoimmune disease really intrigued me. The more I read, the more I felt that I wanted to try eliminating wheat to see if it could help me manage my pain.

"I used to LOVE going for walks. If I walk now, even just for a few miles, I am in so much pain it's just not worth it. What motivates me is to just keep improving, to prove to myself that there's an inner athlete inside of me, a woman who is in control of her destiny and her health, not at the mercy of this chronic muscle and joint pain. If following this lifestyle truly helps diminish some of the chronic pain that I feel, that would mean more than anything to me. That's my goal: to live life to the fullest, to treat my body with respect by exercising regularly and eating foods that nourish it, and to just feel good and pain-free every day."

This is why I tell you about such effects, so that you understand this can and does happen. Don't let it happen to you in your quest for grain-free, fully empowered health.

A WHEAT BELLY HEALTH MAKEOVER

Recognize these essential truths about wheat and grains and you will be empowered in ways and to a degree that you thought unattainable. Because of previous failures, you may have come to believe, for instance, that you would never again achieve high school weight, or fit into a size 8 dress or skinny jeans, or have a flat tummy, or not rely on prescription medications, or simply go about your day unimpaired by stiffness and fatigue. Part of the transformation of the Wheat Belly 10-Day Detox is to start believing again that you can achieve these goals.

My days are packed with hearing the success stories of people who have lost as much as 150 pounds, have dropped from double-digit dress sizes to single digits, are able to stop long lists of prescription drugs, have regained youthful energy, and are earning compliments from friends and family who are convinced they've either discovered the Fountain of Youth or undergone expert plastic surgery without the scars. While the weight loss and youth-restoring effects are indeed wonderful, it's the turnaround in health that is most exciting: No other lifestyle approach has the potential to minimize, even fully reverse, the hundreds of health conditions that the Wheat Belly 10-Day Detox can address.

The full benefits of this lifestyle can only get a powerful start during these first 10 days, with longer periods required, of course, to drop 12 dress sizes, lose 100 pounds, or reverse more complex health conditions. But you will more than likely get a powerful sense of the tidal wave of changes that are going to take place. You will see this reflected, too, in the stories of our detox panelists—the ups, the downs, the tsunami of body changes—as they begin their health-restoring and weight-loss journey.

Weight loss can be achieved by cutting calories and portion sizes (though it is a painful process that requires monumental willpower), counting "points," cutting carbs, and even cutting fat (at least at first). But such weight-loss efforts achieve just that: weight loss, often accompanied by plenty of tears, doubts, cravings, swearing, self-loathing, and temptation. Weight loss can restore limited aspects of health, but it certainly won't reverse unhealthy bowel flora, or provide relief from joint pain or bowel urgency, or reverse inflammatory, autoimmune, or neurological conditions. Losing weight alone is like applying new cosmetics: You may look a little nicer and present a better face to the world, but your underlying health is not improved by a new eye shadow or shade of lipstick.

Let's instead view excess weight not as just excess weight, but as a reflection of disrupted health, an outward sign of hormonal and metabolic signals gone haywire. In other words, if you carry excess weight, look at this no differently than, say, high blood sugar, high blood pressure, high triglycerides, an inflammatory condition, or lupus. They are all abnormal health conditions. Losing weight is just losing weight—that is not what you should be achieving. If that were true, starvation would be a perfect health strategy. You should aim to achieve health; weight loss will follow naturally, effortlessly, without counting calories, without limiting portions, without reducing fat. You are going to experience a

PHILIPPA, 40,
administrative assistant, Virginia

"The way that I felt at 20 versus 40 years old is dramatically different. If I project out another 20 years to 60 years old, I'm not sure how motivated I'll be to stick around. The joint pain and exhaustion could be ridiculous by then. I have to figure out how to feel better.

"I don't want to retire and feel awful. I don't want to shop in the plus sizes. I don't want another 10 years of avoiding family pictures because I'm not comfortable in my own skin. I used to be confident and aggressive. Now I clam up because I feel ugly and weak. I want to play tennis and basketball with my 12-year-old instead of being tired. Why does my desk job exhaust me? It's not normal!

"I HAVE to do this for me."

genuine head-to-toe, inside-and-out body makeover. We will, however, have to talk about carbohydrates, as they have proliferated in modern foods to such an extraordinary degree, thanks to the misguided low-fat message that now determines food manufacturers' product designs.

While banishing all things wheat and grains sounds like an overwhelming process to some, it is readily accomplished once you understand the rules on how to navigate foods. But it doesn't end there. Just as an alcoholic who stops drinking two fifths of bourbon a day on Tuesday is not restored to perfect health by Thursday, or even a year later, so it goes with wheat and grains. There are additional steps you must take to heal the wounds incurred from 10, 20, 40, or more years of their consumption. These further steps are necessary to regain health, reprogramming your body by following this new dietary script. Gastrointestinal, immune, and metabolic health, in particular, require special coddling, even during our rapid-fire 10-day timeline.

Some of you may also want to achieve as much weight loss and health in as short a time as possible (while doing it safely, of course). Perhaps you allowed weight to get far out of control while enduring years of prescription drugs for a variety of health struggles, never once suspecting that your high-fiber breakfast cereal or the drug prescribed for high blood pressure or an allergy was among the culprits causing weight gain.

Upon learning that simple food choices are to blame for starting the entire list of health disruptions, you may now be motivated and excited to reverse this disastrous health mess as fast as possible. But let's be realistic: If you have, say, 150 pounds to lose, it's not going to happen in 10 days. But the health benefits that get jump-started during these initial 10 days, even if the weight loss amounts to no more than 5 pounds, are going to be crucial in setting the stage for future continued success because, remember, you are trying to reestablish health, not just a healthy weight.

PUT ON YOUR BEST PERFUME,
LIGHT SOME CANDLES ...

All right, enough of trying to get you in the mood. Let's get down to business.

I'd like to make one last request before some of the most profound changes in your life get under way. The Wheat Belly 10-Day Detox process is contrary to prevailing nutritional "wisdom" and will cause you to discard most of the ideas about health and nutrition that you may have held for most of your life. This means that you'd do best by starting with a clean slate, free of decades of misinformation and marketing. I'm asking you to open your mind to the possibility that the worldwide epidemic of obesity is not due to new and widespread extremes of gluttony and laziness, that the boom in diabetes should not be blamed on human weakness, that the explosion in autoimmune diseases should not be blown off as inheriting a bad genetic hand, and that the process of detoxification should not involve ingesting juices with magical properties or tubes inserted in uncomfortable places. Be open to the possibility that real answers lie elsewhere and you will be empowered to enjoy the solution.

In the interest of getting you to your goals as quickly and powerfully as possible, I won't dwell anymore on the science or ponder how and why this lifestyle achieves so many goals that previously eluded you. In the rest of the book, we will be concerned with the practical steps that get you to your weight and health goals as quickly, effortlessly, and effectively as possible.

The Wheat Belly 10-Day Detox is a hard-hitting, nononsense, no-romantic-interlude kind of book, an ultra quick-start to a life-changing way of eating, unfettered by the details of the *why* (which, should your curiosity be piqued, can be found in the preceding Wheat Belly books). Be prepared to tighten your belt and to rediscover what freely mobile joints and normal bowel habits feel like and what it means to be clearheaded and energetic while enjoying food like you never have before.

CHAPTER 2

YOUR 10 DAYS START NOW

YOUR 10-DAY COUNTDOWN to a new life that is dramatically different starts *now*.

Sit down, grab a handle, and strap yourself in: You are going for the ride of your life. It will be a roller coaster of emotional and physical turbulence, with a few yelps, nausea, and moments of panic along the way that will land you in a place you likely have not been before—a world of health, single-digit clothes sizes, feeling wonderful, and being the recipient of jealous looks from the perplexed and frustrated grain-eaters around you, as well as of appreciative looks from your partner. This is your ticket to that world.

It may sound like an overused, over-the-top prediction to say that the Wheat Belly 10-Day Detox experience will be life changing, but I assure you it will. It will be as life changing as surviving the throes of adolescence minus the acne and social bumbling, as life changing as having children without the diapers and sleepless nights. I predict that the changes will be so dramatic you will wonder how you managed to endure life before you discovered these answers to your health and weight struggles.

You may come to view your life as pre-detox and post-detox. Those of you who start the process with a health problem or five can typically expect dramatic improvements in health and the way you feel. Even within the first week, joint pains in the fingers and wrists, acid reflux, facial redness and rash, and bowel urgency can disappear, while over the second week and onward energy improves, the belly shrinks visibly, and pain in larger joints like knees and hips can begin to recede. It's not uncommon for health to improve in such a broad front that it's hard to keep up with reducing or eliminating prescription medications. People with high blood pressure or diabetes, in particular, commonly witness marked reductions in blood pressure and blood sugar within days, making it necessary to whittle down medications rapidly (to be discussed).

You may find it helpful to record your experience with this detox, as well as your long-term Wheat Belly journey. Maintaining a journal that chronicles the health and life changes that you undergo can help in the future, when you may start telling yourself things like "My life before Wheat Belly really wasn't that bad," or as memories of your grain-filled tribulations recede (as memories often do), or as friends try to persuade you to go back to the grain dark side. Refer back to your recorded descriptions of the changes you endured, the withdrawal effects, the health transformations you enjoyed, and the improvements in the way you feel, and you will be reminded that you did indeed undergo some dramatic changes and that going back is a really bad idea. Even better, consider also snapping some "before" selfies or find some recent photos of yourself that you can hold up against the "after" pictures. I predict that this graphic record of the changes you are going to experience will astound you with their stark contrast. Include close-up photos of your face, as these will especially highlight the changes you'll experience.

Even people who start this process just to lose a few pounds, but feel pretty good at the start, report that they feel even better after the initial detox, noting that issues they'd come to accept as part of life, such as rashes, foot pain, or mental fog, have disappeared. People will say, "I didn't realize that I really didn't feel that great, but now I feel better than I have in 20 years." In addition to feeling 20 years younger, many actually look 20 years younger.

But I won't kid you: For many people, things may get worse before they get better. The first several days of your detox may be tumultuous, filled with emotional ups and downs and unpleasant experiences. You will see this reflected in the experiences of our detox panelists, including Jennifer, who endured a week of incapacitating fatigue and headaches before she began to emerge. An occasional person will experience transient worsening of chronic joint pain or migraine headaches. It will almost certainly disrupt the routine of your life: You may sleep longer; the dishes and dirty laundry may pile up; the family may be annoyed at your apparent malaise.

Much of this is due to stopping the flow of the unique, only partially digestible proteins in grains (gliadin in wheat, secalin in rye, hordein in barley, zein in corn) that yield the opiates that drive appetite. Yes: Law-abiding, PTA-card-holding mothers and fathers, housewives, teachers, and businesspeople who consume grains are opiate addicts. Casts a whole new light on breakfast cereals with names like Krave, doesn't it? By stopping the flow of grains in your daily diet, you halt the flow of opiates, and an opiate-withdrawal syndrome can result. Unfortunately, for the people who do experience it, there is no way to avoid this phenomenon. There are ways to make the process less unpleasant that we will discuss, but if you are destined to have it, you must go through this process in order to free yourself from the mind-gripping and appetite-magnifying effects of grain-derived opiates. View it as a necessary step to return to health, much as a drug addict must stop injecting or snorting a drug and endure the withdrawal process before life can start anew.

It will be important to recognize withdrawal for what it is and not mistake it for something else. You especially don't want to think, "Gee, my body must be telling me that I need grains." There is no intrinsic need for anything in grains, and there is no deficiency created by removing them, but there is everything to gain by removing them and enduring this withdrawal process.

Of the 10 detox volunteer panelists, by the way, all 10 got to the finish, now sobered by the experience of the withdrawal process, understanding that wheat and grains had been having such a profound effect on their bodies that the process of reversing it was necessary to reclaim control over their lives.

SUSANNE, 51, jewelry designer, Georgia

"My symptoms were joint pain, and they did get worse before they got better. I was very fatigued the first few days, but just took naps and headed to bed early. Drinking more water was a huge help, as well.

"The hardest part about giving up grains is realizing they are everywhere, hidden in everything we eat. Knowing what to look for if you stray from single-ingredient foods is sooo key. It is a new learning curve but very empowering."

The only reason to delay starting your 10-day transformation would be to choose a time without an impending period of high-pressure work or school deadlines or other stressful situations in order to better endure the withdrawal process. It will be especially difficult if, for instance, you have to work 16-hour days for an upcoming deadline while enduring the emotional roller coaster, mental fogginess, nausea, and fatigue of grain withdrawal. It's not much worse than having a bad case of the flu without the nasal stuffiness, except that you are in charge of when you are going to endure it. You might also delay it if you have a major travel obligation coming, such as a family vacation, as it will be best to have your kitchen available to you during this period. Short of these potential disruptive factors in your near future, however, you should brace yourself and just get started now.

But don't delay unnecessarily. Much as you do not want to delay the delivery of a baby at the 9-month mark of pregnancy or the bellyache of an urgent bowel movement triggered by the intestinal irritants of wheat and grains, so you shouldn't allow another moment to pass before you consider beginning your journey.

THE THREE STEPS OF GRAIN DETOX

The Wheat Belly 10-Day Detox begins with the concept that the foods we are told (over and over and over again) should dominate our diet—grains—need to be completely removed in all their varied forms. This is the first big step in taking back control over weight and health. It means removing the appetite-stimulating effects of cookies and bagels, the autoimmune disease–triggering effects of multigrain bread, the behavior-distortion and learning impairment of animal crackers, and the gastrointestinal disruption of breakfast cereals. It may sound drastic, some even say impossible. Others say it will lead to nutrient deficiencies, difficulty navigating social situations, getting kicked out of the country club, friends no longer talking to you, having to take confession with your priest, even malnutrition and disabling deficiencies. None of this is true.

Once you are aware of a few basic ground rules in your newly empowered grain-free life, I predict that you will find this lifestyle entirely manageable, liberating, delicious, and healthy. Yes, there will be efforts that take some getting used to, such as asking waitstaff at restaurants about ingredients in dishes you order, but such efforts are minimal and easily accomplished. And this is what you must do in order to gain extraordinary control over appetite and health.

To make the transition to grain-free living a digestible process for you, even if your life is hectic and crammed with other responsibilities, I've broken it down into three bite-size, grain-free, sugar-free pieces. The three steps to getting started on this lifestyle are:

1. Eliminate all grains.
2. Eat real, single-ingredient foods.
3. Manage carbohydrates.

It's that simple. Yes, there are additional steps to take to regain body-wide health, and we'll discuss them later in the book.

But the effort to convert from an unwitting, helpless, inflamed, weight-accumulating, disease-causing, grain-filled diet to a health-empowering, performance-enhancing, feel-great-again, grain-free diet is just that easy.

When we revert to eating foods that we are adapted to consume (since grains were added only a moment in time ago, speaking anthropologically), there are no concerns about saturated fat or fiber, there is nothing sugared-up, nobody needs to count calories, and there are certainly no products made from grains. We leave behind worries about portion size or overeating. We return to foods that allowed humans to survive and thrive for more than 99 percent of our time on Earth, when being overweight and the diseases of civilization (such as diabetes, hypertension, and autoimmune diseases) were unknown, before we mistakenly turned to grains in desperation as a source of calories when nothing better was available; we used grains then as food to provide sustenance, grow, and reproduce without knowing their enormous long-term health-disrupting impact.

Re-creating such a new, yet really old, pre-grain diet means making allowances for the modern choices we are presented, since we will not be spearing wild boar or digging in the dirt for wild roots. We therefore need to learn how to navigate their closest modern counterparts in places like supermarkets.

We begin with the indispensable, unavoidable, and absolutely necessary first step.

STEP 1: Eliminate All Grains

We start by eliminating the unexpected and surprising source of so many problems: no, not your nitpicky mother-in-law or your spouse's excessive sports TV–watching habits, but grains. It is not uncommon for people to obtain more than half of their daily calories from grains. Eliminating them represents a major disruption of shopping, eating, and cooking habits. But I know of nothing—extreme exercise, prescription drugs, nutritional supplements, cleansing enemas, meditation, a year in a monastery—that can match the benefits of removing these disrupters of health.

Grain elimination is by far the most important step in the detox, because the next few steps will follow this crucial first step naturally. By banishing grains, you eliminate the appetite-stimulating effects of grain-derived opiates, effects that encourage consumption of junk carbohydrates. You will also eliminate gastrointestinal toxins in grains that alter your sense of taste. Minus these effects, your appetite will be reduced, you will spend far less time being hungry (if you are hungry at all), and your sense of taste will be reawakened. You will actually find former goodies no longer good, even sickeningly sweet, and you will enjoy healthy foods more. You will discover, for instance, that Brussels sprouts and blueberries have dimensions of flavor you never experienced before. The physiological changes that you undergo in Step 1 make the two subsequent steps of your detox easier.

Let me be absolutely clear on this: Eliminate all grains. I don't mean cut back. I don't mean every day except Friday. I don't mean only at home, while drifting back to grain-consuming ways at restaurants or friends' homes. Even a little compromise can completely block your success, halt the detoxification process, sustain the opiate addictive and appetite-stimulating effects, and continue to cultivate inflammation. So when I say "eliminate all grains," I mean 100 percent without compromise, no matter where you are, what other people say, or what day of the week it is.

This first step is unavoidable. You cannot succeed in this lifestyle without this critical first step and going the full distance with it, else none of the other steps will follow or achieve the effects you desire. So let's talk about how you can accomplish this all-important first step and banish all grains from your life.

Start with a Grain-Free Kitchen

I recommend starting this lifestyle by creating a grain-free kitchen: Establish a grain-free zone that includes your refrigerator, pantry, and cabinet shelves purged of all foods made with grains. Grocery stores, fast-food joints, and schools may be stocked top to bottom with them, but your personal kitchen will be a grain-free safe zone, a haven for healthy eating.

Start by removing all obvious sources of wheat flour such as bread, rolls, doughnuts, pasta, cookies, cake, pretzels, crackers, pancake mix, breakfast cereals, bread crumbs, and bagels. Toss out all the coupons you've set aside to save a few dollars on delivery pizza or bakery items. Then remove all bottled, canned, packaged, and frozen processed foods with wheat among the ingredients. Check the labels for wheat in all its various forms, some of which are obvious and others that are not so obvious, with names such as modified food starch, panko, seitan, and bran. (See Appendix B for a list of hidden grain sources and names.)

Tackle barley-containing foods next. This includes any food with malt listed on the label, as well as barley itself. (Beer and some other alcoholic beverages have grain issues, but we will discuss this in Appendix B.) Any foods made with rye, such as rye breads and rye crackers, should all go, too.

Now remove all obvious sources of corn, such as corn on the cob, canned corn, corn chips, tacos, and grits, as well as processed packaged foods made with obvious and not-so-obvious corn ingredients such as hydrolyzed cornflour and polenta (also listed in Appendix B).

Other grains, such as oats, rice, millet, sorghum, amaranth, and teff, are usually listed by their real names; purge the kitchen of these foods.

Why are grains found in so many processed foods? Sometimes

they are there for legitimate reasons, such as to improve texture and taste or to thicken. But grains are also a way to bulk up a product inexpensively, causing you to believe that a frozen pizza is a bargain. In other words, grains are cheap filler. It is a way to feed people cheaply with plates piled high and appetites satisfied—at least for a few minutes, until they are hungry again. Note that fast-food restaurants are monuments to the use of cheap filler, so it is very difficult (impossible in some outlets) to navigate a meal free of them in such places.

But I believe that grains are present in nearly all processed foods for reasons beyond cheap filler. The dirty little secret is that grains increase food consumption by yielding opiates that increase appetite, adding an average of 400 more calories per person, per day, every day (averaging the food intake of everybody: adults, infants, and children). It's not uncommon for grains to provoke consumption of 1,000 or more additional calories per day in an adult. Top off processed foods with high-fructose corn syrup, a highly processed derivative of corn, with its low-cost, intense sweetness, and you increase the expectation of sweetness and further amp up appetite in the consuming public, further increasing our desire for other sweet, processed foods. (Grain-free people, by the way, find the taste and sweetness of high-fructose corn syrup overwhelming, something you will lose all desire for, another reflection of sharpened taste.) As a consumer of "healthy whole grains," you were doomed from the start, but now you know.

Just as there is no way to make a cigarette healthy, there is no way to salvage any of the grain products you had in your pantry or refrigerator. Toss them in the trash, give them to charity, use them for compost or cat litter, but get rid of them. This removes the temptation to "just have one cracker" or think that "just one bite won't hurt" or try to avoid waste. We will discuss why it is so important to not allow this to happen and avoid the reactivation of appetite and addictive behavior, as well as triggering reexposure

Start Your Grain-Free Wheat Belly 10-Day Detox

Clear your kitchen of all obvious wheat and grain sources

- Wheat-based products: bread, rolls, breakfast cereals, pasta, orzo, bagels, muffins, pancakes and pancake mixes, waffles, doughnuts, pretzels, cookies, crackers

- Bulgur and triticale (both related to wheat)

- Barley products: barley, barley breads, soups with barley, vinegars with barley malt

- Rye products: rye bread, pumpernickel bread, crackers

- All corn products: corn, cornflour, cornmeal products (chips, tacos, tortillas), grits, polenta, sauces or gravies thickened with cornflour, corn syrup, high-fructose corn syrup, breakfast cereals

- Rice products: white rice, brown rice, wild rice, rice cakes, breakfast cereals

- Oat products: oatmeal, oat bran, oat cereals

reactions that involve bloating, diarrhea, joint pain, and other annoying, even painful, effects. Making the break abruptly and cleanly is very important for success. If you are unable to completely purge your kitchen of grain products because, say, a spouse or other family member refuses to go along with your lifestyle change, make it clear that you are going to have food set aside to suit your new eating choices. (In Chapter 7, we will discuss how to quietly and cleverly convert such people over to your way of living. It can be done.)

There is no need for a panic attack, worrying that you will never have a pizza, muffin, or piece of cheesecake again. You will, though we will re-create them using truly healthy ingredients

- Amaranth

- Teff

- Millet

- Sorghum

Then eliminate hidden sources by reading labels

Eliminate hidden sources of grains by avoiding the processed foods that fill the inner aisles of the grocery store. Almost all of these are thickened, flavored, or textured with grain products, or grains are added as cheap filler and/or appetite stimulants.

Living without grains means avoiding foods that you never thought contained grains, such as seasoning mixes bulked up with cornflour, canned and dry soup mixes with wheat flour, soy sauce, frozen dinners with wheat-containing gravy and muffins, and all breakfast cereals, hot and cold. (You will find lists of the hidden aliases for wheat and corn, in particular, that can be found in so many processed foods in Appendix B.)

This does not mean you will never have a crunchy breakfast "cereal" again or a salad topped with delicious dressing. You will learn to either make your own versions with no unhealthy grains to booby-trap your lifestyle or to identify the brands that have no grains or other unhealthy ingredients added.

that will not cause weight gain or reverse the health benefits you've worked to achieve. (You will be introduced to these in the 10-Day Menu Plan in Chapter 5.)

Go Grain-Free Shopping

You have purged your kitchen of grain-containing foods and need to restock with new, healthy, grain-free alternatives. Go to the supermarket or the stores where you shop for meat, vegetables, and other foods. (Some of our detox panelists observed that they needed to shop at more than one store in their neighborhood to find all the starting ingredients.) One observation you are sure to make as you remove all grains from your life and carefully examine labels is, "This is impossible. Grains are in everything!"

Indeed, grains—especially wheat and corn—are in salad dressings, seasoning mixes, licorice, frozen dinners, breakfast cereals, canned soups, dried soup mixes, rotisserie chickens, soft drinks, whiskies, beers, prescription drugs, shampoos, conditioners, lipstick, chewing gum, and even the adhesive in envelopes. Wheat and corn are in virtually every processed food on grocery store shelves and in many cosmetics and toiletries, as ubiquitous as (how can I resist?) white on rice. (By the way, steal a look at the contents of other shoppers' grocery carts and you will be amazed at the number of foods that contain wheat and grains. You'll be hard-pressed to find foods that don't contain them.)

It also means bearing some greater up-front grocery costs, since you are restocking much of your kitchen with new foods. Don't be fooled, though: The increased costs of following the Wheat Belly lifestyle will not continue forever. It's just part of getting started. Recall that, as you progress in your wheat- and grain-free lifestyle, food and calorie consumption will drop naturally. If your family follows suit, multiply the reduced food intake by the number of family members, and it all adds up (in the experience of most people) to reduced long-term costs or no increase—making no dent in your monthly food budget, despite getting rid of all the foods made with cheap filler and replacing them with higher-quality substitutes.

Of the 60,000 or so processed food products that pack the shelves of the average supermarket, your options will be whittled down to about 1,000, but you should never feel deprived. You will discover that the foods you've eliminated are nearly all variations on the same processed food theme: wheat flour, cornflour, sugar, high-fructose corn syrup, and food coloring, whether it was breakfast cereal, a pop-in-the-toaster convenience breakfast, frozen waffles, low-calorie frozen dinners, or crackers. They're all cheap filler in the modern diet, dolled up with the glitz of modern marketing.

Start by not shopping for obvious sources of wheat, corn, and other grains and avoid the bread aisle, the bakery, frozen food freezers, the breakfast cereal aisle, and the internal aisles stocked with packaged foods. Confine your shopping to the produce section, the butcher counter, and the dairy refrigerator; venture into the inner aisles only for spices, nuts and seeds, laundry detergent and other household supplies, and dog or cat food (though you might consider looking for grain-free pet food, as well). You may wish to consult the day-by-day shopping list for the 10-Day Menu Plan in Appendix A to be sure you have the ingredients on hand to create the plan's recipes.

You are aiming to achieve a diet filled with foods that are least processed. The most confident means of avoiding foods with grains is to choose foods that are naturally grain-free, such as vegetables, eggs, olives, and meats. That points us toward a solution, a policy that helps you easily navigate your new grain-less life: Avoid processed foods that bear labels and return to real, unprocessed, naturally grain-free, single-ingredient foods without labels.

STEP 2: Choose Real, Single-Ingredient Foods

An avocado, intact in its skin, can be chosen with confidence, as no food manufacturer added grains to it. Eggs in their shell likewise. In other words, foods left more or less intact and unmodified by a food manufacturer should top your list of foods to choose from that are safe for your empowering grain-free lifestyle. Avocados and whole eggs are real—not fake, multiple-ingredient marketing conceptions of some food manufacturer—and there's no chance of exposure to grains, added sugars, high-fructose corn syrup, hydrogenated oils, or other no-no's.

You will find the majority of real, single-ingredient foods in the produce section, butcher counter, and dairy refrigerator. Depending on the layout of your supermarket, you may have to venture into those hazardous internal aisles for some of your baking supplies, spices, and nuts, but do so while ignoring all the packaged, processed, glitzy, eye-catching products.

Avoiding foods with labels simplifies the task of label reading. Cucumbers, spinach, and pork chops, for example, don't come with labels (except to display weight and date). Avoiding labels means you'll be buying foods in their basic, least modified forms. Sure, the pork chops were sliced from a larger piece of the meat from the animal, but they should not have been changed in any other way.

This simple policy of choosing real, single-ingredient foods has served prior Wheat Belly followers well, served our detox panelists well, and will serve you well, particularly as you are learning to navigate this lifestyle at the start.

Choosing real, single-ingredient foods that are nourishing and don't yield land mines in your Wheat Belly 10-Day Detox means enjoying unlimited quantities of the following:

VEGETABLES. Enjoy all the fresh or frozen veggies you want, except for potatoes (see "Step 3: Manage Carbohydrates" on page 37—unless you're consuming the potatoes raw, as suggested in Chapter 4). Explore the wonderful range of choices: spinach, chard, kale, broccoli, broccolini, collard greens, lettuces, peppers, onions, mushrooms, Brussels sprouts, courgettes, squash, and so on. It may also be time to revisit vegetables you didn't previously like because of the change in taste perception you will undergo when grain-free. Don't be surprised if the Brussels sprouts you once despised now become your favorite. Minimize reliance on canned vegetables, especially tomatoes, due to bisphenol A, an endocrine-disrupting chemical, in the can's lining.

MEATS. Choose from beef, pork, lamb, fish, chicken, turkey, buffalo, ostrich, and wild game. Consider pasture-/grass-fed, free-range, and organic sources whenever possible to minimize exposure to antibiotic residues, hormones, and other contaminants, as well as to do your part in encouraging a return to more humane livestock practices. There is no need to look for lean cuts; look for fatty cuts, often less expensive and full of the fats you need that facilitate success in this lifestyle. And try to overcome the modern aversion to organ meats, such as liver, heart, and tongue, the most nutritious components of all, especially liver and heart. Uncured liver sausage or ground liver added to meat loaf are easy ways to resume organ consumption. Only over the last 50 years have people developed an aversion to organ meats. Get over it: Have some liver. (Just as with humans, if an animal was raised in contaminated circumstances, the meat and organs will be contaminated likewise, so look for pasture-fed, organic sources here, as well.) Save bones in the freezer to make soups and stocks, excellent for joint, hair, and nail health.

EGGS. Eggs are little powerhouses of nutrition and are an important part of a successful grain-free lifestyle. We do not limit eggs, since the alarms over the potential cardiovascular risks of eggs have been confidently debunked. Choose free-range, organic sources whenever possible or, even better, purchase them from a local source. If you are allergic to eggs from chickens, consider goose, duck, ostrich, or quail eggs, if available.

RAW OR DRY-ROASTED NUTS AND SEEDS. Almonds, walnuts, pecans, hazelnuts, pistachios, Brazil nuts, macadamia nuts, pumpkin seeds, sunflower seeds, sesame seeds, flaxseeds, and chia seeds are all great choices, as are dry-roasted peanuts (though they're really a low-carbohydrate legume, not a nut). Avoid nuts roasted in unhealthy oils, such as hydrogenated cottonseed or hydrogenated soybean oil, as well as wheat flour, cornflour, maltodextrin, or sugar used to coat them. Should you choose roasted, none of these unhealthy oils or other ingredients should be listed. Cashews are the one nut that should be limited, as they are among the most carbohydrate-rich of nuts; consume lightly and use the carbohydrate management method discussed below.

FATS AND OILS. Choose coconut, palm, extra-virgin olive, extra-light olive, macadamia, avocado, flaxseed, and walnut oils, as well as organic butter and ghee. Don't be afraid of saving the oils from bacon, beef, and pork. You can also purchase lard and tallow, but make sure they are not hydrogenated. Minimize use of polyunsaturated oils (corn, safflower, mixed vegetable, and sunflower). Avoid hydrogenated or partially hydrogenated oils completely.

CHEESES. Purchase real cultured cheeses only (not single-slice processed cheese), preferably organic and full fat, not skim or reduced fat. The cheese-making process minimizes the undesirable aspects of dairy (such as whey and unhealthy forms of casein). Be careful with blue cheese, Gorgonzola, and Roquefort, which are occasionally sources of wheat.

BEVERAGES. Drink water (squeeze in some lemon or lime or keep a filled water pitcher in the refrigerator with a few slices of cucumber, kiwifruit, mint leaves, or orange), teas (black, green, or white), infusions (teas brewed from other leaves, herbs, flowers, and fruits), unsweetened almond milk, unsweetened coconut milk (the carton variety from the dairy refrigerator), unsweetened hemp milk, and coffee. Sip the Coconut Electrolyte Replacement Water (page 152) as is or on ice. Avoid sodas and fruit drinks, even the sugar-free ones as they are typically sweetened with aspartame and have been associated with weight gain and unhealthy changes in bowel flora.

MISCELLANEOUS. Look for guacamole, hummus, pesto, tapenades, olives, and unsweetened condiments, such as mayonnaise, mustard, ketchup without high-fructose corn syrup, and oil-based salad dressings without high-fructose corn syrup, sugar, dextrose, or cornflour.

ALCOHOL. It is best to refrain from alcohol or keep it to a bare minimum (no more than one glass per day) during your detox. If you wish to keep some on hand, though, consider wine (the drier, the better); non-grain vodka (Cîroc, Chopin, others); rum; tequila; brandies and cognacs; and non-grain or gluten-free beers

(Redbridge, Green's, Bard's, and others). Note that beers, in particular, can have small quantities of grain residues, even if gluten-free, and have potential for excessive carbohydrates, so go very lightly with them; one 12-ounce serving approaches your carbohydrate limit, so never have more than one serving. (There is a more detailed listing of safe alcoholic beverages in Appendix B.)

STEP 3: Manage Carbohydrates

The third step in the Wheat Belly 10-Day Detox is to manage carbohydrates, even beyond those found in grains, as they are the darlings of the processed food industry—cheap, tasty filler that contributes to dietary helplessness and health distortions. Carbohydrates provoke blood sugar and insulin and slow, even stop, your weight loss and health efforts. Properly managing these foods allows you to squeeze additional benefits from the power of your grain-free nutritional program. It will supercharge weight loss and allow you to gain further control over metabolic disturbances, such as high blood sugars, fatty liver, triglycerides, blood pressure, and needing to shop in plus-size aisles.

We follow this simple rule: Never exceed 15 grams net carbohydrates per meal or per 6-hour (digestive) period. We calculate net carbs by the following simple equation:

NET CARBS = TOTAL CARBS – FIBER

Because most of your foods will not come with labels or nutritional panels, you will need a resource to look up the composition of various foods, such as an inexpensive handbook with tables of the nutritional content of foods. (Find these in the reference section of your local library or bookstore, often for less than $10.) There are also several terrific smartphone apps useful for this purpose. (Search for "nutritional analysis" in your application source.) In addition, there are many Web sites that list nutritional analyses of foods. Look up total carbohydrate and fiber content of the food in question, make the simple calculation, and you have net carbohydrate content.

Nothing matches the power of eliminating grains to reduce inflammation, recover gastrointestinal health, reduce appetite, and drop weight. But banishing all grains while feasting on a bag of potato chips or downing three cans of sugary cola every day can still trip up health and weight. Carbohydrate management helps you sidestep problem sources and compound the benefits begun with grain elimination. And because diabetes and over-weight are concerns for so many people at the start of their detox, this step is also necessary to take control of these modern epidemic conditions.

Carb management is easier than it sounds once grains have been eliminated, even for people who begin this process with a sweet tooth. Recall that ridding your life of grain-derived opiates reduces appetite and reawakens taste, including heightening sensitivity to sweetness. The desire for sweet snacks diminishes or disappears, and goodies you formerly thought were irresistible will taste sickeningly sweet. Addiction to milk chocolate, gummy candy, or other junk indulgences will go the way of padded shoulders and harem pants. Good riddance.

We also do not use the misleading fiction of the glycemic index or glycemic load. (See "The Fairy Tale of Glycemic Index" on page 40.) Choosing low-glycemic index foods, for instance, will trigger blood sugar and insulin to high levels, cause weight gain, and prevent the health benefits of this lifestyle—virtually no different than high-glycemic index foods. Don't fall for the health and weight booby-trap of glycemic index.

Your efforts to manage carbohydrates will limit rises in blood sugar. Contrary to conventional advice from most doctors (who typically advise that blood sugars should not exceed 11 mmol/L after a meal, a level associated with astounding levels of weight gain and health impairment), adhering to our 15 g net carb cutoff keeps blood sugars at or below 6 mmol/L at all times, including blood sugar after eating a meal. In other words, we aim to never allow blood sugar to rise over the level present prior to the meal.

If you have diabetes or prediabetes and start with higher-than-normal blood sugars, this approach will prevent additional rises in blood sugar with meals and allow even future fasting blood sugars to drop over time. We therefore work to keep blood sugars at healthy levels when you rise in the morning; before and after breakfast, lunch, and dinner; before bedtime; when you wear open-toed shoes, high heels, or go barefoot; as well as all other times of the day.

By avoiding spikes in blood sugar, insulin release is minimally triggered. Insulin is the root of much dietary and metabolic evil; it is a hormone that causes weight gain and blocks mobilization of stored fat from fat cells. Not triggering insulin allows the opposite to occur: mobilization of fat and weight loss from fat cells. Over time, insulin resistance is reduced, allowing weight loss to progress further. Along with it, inflammation, fatty liver, blood pressure, high triglycerides, inappropriate questions about your baby's due date, and other distortions all strike a retreat.

It is important that, as part of your carbohydrate management effort, you do not limit fats or oils. In the Wheat Belly 10-Day Detox, there are no limits on fat or oil intake, provided you choose your sources wisely. It means you should enjoy the fat on meats, just like your grandparents did. Don't buy meats lean; buy fatty cuts. Don't trim the fat off beef, pork, lamb, or poultry; eat it. Eat dark poultry meat, as well as white. In addition:

- Save fats from cooking beef, pork, and bacon in a container and refrigerate to use as cooking oil.
- Save the bones (or buy them from a butcher) to make soup or stock and don't skim off the fat when it cools.
- Consider enjoying bone marrow.

(continued on page 42)

The Fairy Tale of Glycemic Index

The Wheat Belly 10-Day Detox is a hard-hitting natural approach for gaining incredible control over weight and health in as short a time as possible. There are no fictions or fairy tales here. But some popular nutritional fairy tales could confuse you or undo the benefits you are trying to achieve. The concept of glycemic index (GI) is one good example: a fictional notion that, if believed like a fairy tale, could have you kissing frogs to make princes.

GI assigns values to foods that describe how high blood sugar climbs over 90 minutes after consuming that food compared to glucose. The GI of a pork chop? Zero: no impact on blood sugar. Three scrambled eggs? Also zero. A plate of kalamata olives and big wedge of feta cheese? Zero again. A zero glycemic index applies to all other meats, fats, oils, most nuts, cheeses, mushrooms, and nonstarchy vegetables. Eat any of these foods and blood sugar won't budge and insulin will not be provoked beyond a minimal level.

While there is really nothing wrong with the concept of GI or the related concept of glycemic load (GL), which factors in quantity of food, the problem lies in how values for GI and GL are interpreted. Standard practice is to (arbitrarily) break GI levels down into high GI (70 or greater), moderate GI (56 to 69), and low GI (55 or less), while GL is broken down into high GL (20 or greater), moderate GL (11 to 19), and low GL (10 or less).

Can you be a little bit pregnant? Can you have a little nuclear war? The same applies to GI: There should be no "low" or "high" distinguished by such small differences. All GI levels are associated with blood sugars that are too high if weight loss and ideal metabolic health are your goals. Applying the flawed logic of the GI, cornflakes, puffed rice, and pretzels have high GIs (above 70), while whole grain bread, oatmeal, and rice have low GIs, resulting in the conventional advice to includes lots of these low-GI foods in your diet.

A typical nondiabetic person who consumes 125 g (4½ oz) of oats—a low-GI food—in 120 ml (4 fl oz) cup of milk without added sugar will experience a blood sugar level in the neighborhood of 9 mmol/L. This is a high level that provokes the weight-loss blocking effect of insulin, not to mention also triggering (over time) adrenal disruption, cataract formation, damage to joint cartilage, hypertension, heart disease, and neurological deterioration or dementia when provoked repeatedly, as with oatmeal for breakfast every morning. A blood sugar of 10 mmol/L may not be as high as, say, the 10 mmol/L that occurs after consuming a high-GI food, such as a bowl of cornflakes or puffed rice cereal. But it is still high enough to provoke all the destructive effects of high blood sugar.

Low GI would therefore be more accurately labeled as "less-high" GI. Even better, we could just recognize that any GI above zero or low single-digit values should be regarded as high.

The concept of glycemic load that factors in portion size is no better. Under this system, the GL of cornflakes is 23, the GL of oatmeal is 13, and the GL of whole wheat bread is 10, once again lulling you into thinking that foods like oatmeal and whole wheat bread don't raise blood sugar. But they do. Foods like oats and whole wheat bread don't have low GLs; they have less high GLs.

Is there a value that better predicts whether there will be a blood sugar rise? Yes: grams of carbohydrates. Specifically, net grams of carbohydrates obtained by subtracting fiber (since fiber, while included in the total carbohydrates value on nutritional panels, is not digested to sugar):

NET CARBOHYDRATES = TOTAL CARBOHYDRATES – FIBER

If you were to test blood sugars with a fingerstick glucose meter 30 to 60 minutes after consuming a food (when peak blood sugar usually occurs, not 2 hours as advised by physicians for diabetic blood sugar control), you would see that it takes most of us 15 g net carbohydrates before blood sugars rise, regardless of whether they are high-, medium-, or low-GI. We have based all Wheat Belly 10-Day Detox dietary choices and recipes on this limit.

Let's dash another fairy tale commonly offered by the dietary community that can trip up your weight-loss efforts. They often tell us that if a high-GI food is consumed with added proteins, fats, or fiber, the glycemic effect will be reduced. As often occurs in the fictional tales of nutrition, this is an example of something being less bad but not necessarily good. A typical blood sugar after consuming two slices of multigrain bread on an empty stomach might be 10 mmol/L—high enough to provoke insulin, cortisol, insulin resistance, visceral fat accumulation, and inflammation. Consume two slices of multigrain bread with some slices of turkey, mayonnaise, lettuce, and tomatoes, and blood sugar will be around 9 mmol/L—better, yes, but still pretty high.

Less bad is not necessarily good. The wolf can wear Grandma's nightie, but he's still a big, bad, ugly wolf.

- Don't limit egg consumption. Have a three-egg omelet, for instance, with lots of extra-virgin olive oil, pesto, or olive oil–soaked sun-dried tomatoes.
- Use the oils listed above generously in every dish possible.

If you are worried about your cholesterol, know that the majority of people will experience a reduction in the LDL (bad) cholesterol with this lifestyle, along with plummeting triglycerides and a rise in healthy HDL. Eating fats and oils normalizes these predictors of cardiovascular risk. (A full discussion of the why behind these changes, and why and how a low-fat diet ruins health and booby-traps cardiovascular risk, can be found in both the original *Wheat Belly* and in *Wheat Belly Total Health*.)

REBECCA, 44, sales, Connecticut

"Funny: 8 nights with no binge eating and I forgot that for the past 8 years I have binged before going to bed—my biggest demon. I once read that this lady turned her kitchen faucet on so no one would hear her going in the freezer with a spoon to get ice cream. I couldn't believe someone else did that! Wow! This was an addiction, and following the guidelines of Dr. Davis worked. For once I didn't have to pretend to myself that I wasn't starving. Once I gave him my full trust in the process, I upped my fat intake and that was my saving grace."

If we are going to increase our intake of fats and oils, it also means avoiding foods labeled "low-fat" or "nonfat." These terms mean high carbohydrate and high sugar and also serve as buzzwords for grains. Yes, conventional notions of healthy foods with reduced fat have not just wasted our time, but disposed of any control we may have hoped for in weight and health. Have nothing to do with them. If you consume dairy products, for instance, pour the fat-free, 1%, or 2% milk down the drain and go for the full fat or cream. No light coconut milk; we want the thickest, fattiest variety.

We also avoid hydrogenated fats, or trans fats, a common ingredient in processed foods, especially grain-based foods, as they contribute to heart disease, hypertension, and diabetes. Margarine is the worst, made with vegetable oils hydrogenated to yield a solid stick or tub form. Many processed foods, from cookies to sandwich spreads, contain hydrogenated oils and should be avoided for this and other reasons. Use real organic butter or ghee instead (if you include dairy).

Despite our embrace of fats and oils, you should not interpret this to mean that foods deep-fried in oils are healthy. They are not. But it's not so much the fat as the high-temperature reactions that occur in deep-fried foods, even healthy foods, especially if polyunsaturated oils like corn are used. Because of the health-impairing effects of the by-products from high-temperature cooking, we avoid or at least minimize any food that is deep-fried.

There are a few additional tips that are useful for managing carbohydrate intake.

ABSOLUTELY AVOID GLUTEN-FREE FOODS MADE WITH CORN-FLOUR, RICE FLOUR, TAPIOCA STARCH, OR POTATO FLOUR. These are the four ingredients most commonly used in gluten-free processed foods. They are awful for health and will completely shut down any hope of weight loss, often resulting in outright, sometimes outrageous, weight gain and inflammation. Managing carbohydrates to improve control over metabolism and health means 100 percent avoidance of these terrible products marketed to an unsuspecting public thinking they are eating healthy by avoiding gluten.

Nothing raises blood sugar higher than the gluten-free junk carbohydrates in, say, gluten-free multigrain bread or gluten-free pasta—higher than even table sugar. Blood sugar that results from eating two slices of whole grain gluten-free bread made with potato flour, rice flour, and millet can easily top 10 mmol/L (in those without diabetes) over the first hour after consumption, regardless of the mayonnaise, meat, cheese, or other foods in the

Important: If You Start with Diabetes ...

If you are injecting insulin or taking certain diabetes drugs, precautions will be necessary to avoid the potential danger of hypoglycemia (blood sugars lower than 4 mmol/L) and, less commonly, diabetic ketoacidosis, if you have diabetes associated with inadequate pancreatic insulin production. There are also the uninformed objections of many doctors who have come to believe that diabetes is incurable, irreversible, and a diagnosis for life—not true in the majority of cases of type 2 diabetes.

Anyone taking insulin injections in any form will need to reduce the dosage in order to follow this lifestyle without experiencing hypoglycemia. An immediate need to reduce insulin by half is typical. Ideally, this is undertaken with the assistance of a health care provider with experience in helping patients reduce or eliminate their diabetes. This almost always means identifying a new practitioner, as the one who prescribed the insulin for type 2 diabetes in the first place is likely a member of the "diabetes is incurable and irreversible" school, not recognizing that insulin injections are a weight gain drug.

I cannot stress enough that hypoglycemia must be avoided, even if higher blood sugars result temporarily (though ideally kept below 11 mmol/L throughout this process). Other medications, especially oral agents glyburide, glipizide, and glimepiride, can cause dangerous hypoglycemia. For this reason, many people eliminate these oral drugs or reduce doses, even if it means a temporary increase in blood sugars. As blood sugars trend

sandwich. There are indeed some food producers who have developed gluten-free and grain-free products without junk carb ingredients that do not raise blood sugar and so are safe, but they remain in the minority.

LIMIT FRUIT. Adhere to our carb management cutoff and limit yourself to no more than 15 g net carbohydrates per meal. Choose fruit with the least carbohydrate content and greatest nutritional value. From best to worst, choose from: berries of all varieties, cherries, citrus, apples, nectarines, peaches, and melons. 80 g (3 oz) of blueberries, for example, contains 15 g downward, you'll need to further reduce medications. If, for instance, you have fasting blood sugars of 6 mmol/L or less, it is essential to reduce or eliminate a medication.

For people with type 1 diabetes and the uncommon latent autoimmune diabetes of adulthood (LADA) associated with inadequate insulin production, the need for insulin is lifelong and cannot be stopped. Insulin dose, however, as well as the need for oral diabetes medications and drugs for hypertension, inflammation, and other phenomena, can all be reduced dramatically, but anyone with these conditions will always be dependent on insulin. The reduced need for drugs and insulin still greatly reduces risk of long-term diabetic complications.

Because of the complexity of these responses, you should ideally work with a health care provider adept at navigating such issues. Be aware that most doctors and diabetes educators have no idea whatsoever how to do this and will tell you that, once you have type 2 diabetes, you will always have it because that's what the drug industry tells them, or that diet doesn't matter with type 1 diabetes. They may warn you that trying to get rid of type 2 diabetes is dangerous, unproductive, and falsely raises hope. At the very least, you want a doctor who will work with you.

Getting rid of diabetes or minimizing its expression is like getting rid of cancer: It's a really big deal for long-term health. Thankfully, more and more health care providers are seeing through the propaganda of the drug industry and are rejecting the awful advice of the agencies that have contributed to the diabetes epidemic.

total carbohydrates and 3 g fiber = 12 g net carbohydrates. This meets the 15 g or less net carbs limit (but don't forget to factor in other foods you consume along with the blueberries, as it all adds up).

Minimize (ripe) bananas, pineapples, mangoes, and grapes, and when you eat them, do so only in small quantities, since their sugar content is similar to that of candy. A medium 7-inch banana, for example, contains 27 g total carbohydrates and 3 g fiber: 27 − 3 = 24 g net carbohydrates. 80 g (3 oz) of (unsweetened) pineapple chunks contains 20 g total carbs and 1 g fiber = 19 g net carbs. Both the full ripe banana and the 80 g (3 oz) of pineapple chunks are too much and enough to turn off all weight loss and actually begin to trigger some weight gain.

An exception to fruit guidelines are avocados, which are high in fats, rich in potassium, wonderfully filling, and low in net carbs (3 g per avocado).

AVOID FRUIT JUICES. As with fruit, be very careful with fruit juices. You'd do best to avoid juices altogether. If you must drink fruit juice (such as pomegranate or cranberry juice for health benefits), drink only real, 100 percent juice (not fruit "drinks" made with high-fructose corn syrup and little juice) and only in minimal quantities (no more than 55–110 ml (2–4 fl oz) per meal), as the sugar content is too high. One 240 ml (8 fl oz) glass of orange juice, which dominates the breakfast habits of many people who think they are consuming something healthy, contains more than 6 teaspoons of sugar, or 26 g net carbs.

LIMIT DAIRY PRODUCTS. Have no more than 1 serving per day of milk, cottage cheese, or unsweetened yogurt (preferably full fat, if you can find it). Remember: Fat is not the problem. We limit dairy because of the lactose sugar content and the peculiar ability of the whey protein to provoke insulin, which can impair weight loss and encourage insulin resistance, not to mention issues such as estrogen content, bovine growth hormone and antibiotic residues, and potential adverse effects of the casein protein.

Organic, full-fat cheese, full-fat cream cheese, and organic butter and ghee are the least problematic forms of dairy. Organic production avoids growth hormone and minimizes antibiotics, and the culturing process to make cheese reduces lactose and whey, as well as the content of dangerous forms of casein. These products can therefore be safely consumed more liberally, provided you don't have a specific intolerance to one or more dairy components.

LIMIT LEGUMES, COOKED POTATOES, SWEET POTATOES, AND YAMS. Here is where carbohydrate counting can be put to work, keeping intake to no higher than 15 g net carbs per meal. In general, it means eating no more than ¼ of a tea cup of any of these foods per meal. Including some of these foods can be important, however, as they benefit bowel flora, especially raw white potatoes (see the discussion in Chapter 4).

INDULGE IN THE DARKEST CHOCOLATES. Chocolates that are at least 70 percent cocoa, preferably 85 percent or higher, easily fit into your regimen. Count net carbohydrates: the delicious Ghirardelli Intense Dark 86% Cocoa chocolate bar, for instance, contains 15 g total carbs, 5 g fiber (lots of fiber in dark chocolate) = 10 g net carbs in 4 squares (45 g) of chocolate, which is half of the entire 75 g (3 oz) bar, more than enough to satisfy even the most serious chocolate habit. Remember: Wheat and grain elimination amplifies your sense of taste and sweetness so that, even if you previously found dark chocolate to be bitter and not sweet enough, you will now appreciate how delicious it is without the taste distortion of grains. And go ahead: Dip your chocolate into natural peanut butter or almond butter.

BE AWARE OF SAFE VS. UNSAFE SWEETENERS. We have to be picky with our choice of sweeteners, as there are benign sweeteners that we will be using in some of our recipes—cookies, muffins, and pies—and there are destructive sweeteners that impair weight loss and pose other undesirable effects. You need to avoid foods sweetened with the sugar alcohols sorbitol, mannitol, lactitol, or maltitol, as they act much like sugar and cause diarrhea and bloating. Also avoid sucralose, saccharine, and aspartame as there is a theory that they result in unhealthy changes in bowel flora. We will also strictly avoid fructose-containing sweeteners: sucrose (table sugar, which is 50 percent fructose), high-fructose corn syrup, agave nectar (90 percent fructose), coconut sugar, and other sugars marketed as "natural." Some people use honey and maple syrup, as they are natural sources of sugar, but both are high in fructose and should be used sparingly (never more than 1 to 2 teaspoons per serving).

Among the safest sweeteners are pure liquid or powdered ste-via; stevia with inulin but not maltodextrin; monk fruit (also known as luo han guo); and two safe naturally occurring sugar alcohols, erythritol and xylitol. (Be careful with xylitol around dogs, as it is toxic to them.) An occasional person will experience triggering of their sweet tooth with these sweeteners, leading to cravings for other sweet foods, but it is uncommon. Inulin is safe and has a light sweetness and even provides benefits to bowel flora.

A FEW ADDITIONAL STEPS
FOR YOUR WHEAT BELLY DETOX

In the age of modern mass-produced commercial foods, it helps to be aware of several other important issues in order to maxi-mize health. While many of these problems are solved by simply choosing real, single-ingredient foods least manipulated by food manufacturers, there are some foods that, by necessity, are pro-cessed to some degree. We therefore need to navigate carefully to avoid getting tripped up.

MEATS SHOULD BE UNCURED AND UNPROCESSED AND SHOULD NOT CONTAIN SODIUM NITRITE. Sausage, pepperoni, bacon, salami, and other processed meats often contain the color-fixing chemi-cal sodium nitrite. Upon cooking, sodium nitrite reacts with amino acids in meat, yielding nitrosamines that have been linked to gastrointestinal cancers. You should look for meats labeled "uncured" and without sodium nitrite listed on the label (not to be confused with nitrates). Of course, also make sure processed meats contain no wheat, cornflour, or other hidden grains, particularly lunchmeats, sausage, and deli meats.

CHOOSE ORGANIC DAIRY PRODUCTS. Because many commer-cial, high-volume dairies milk pregnant cows throughout preg-nancy (rather than the more limited milking period practiced by organic farmers), products made from this milk contain more estrogen. Minimize this problem by choosing dairy products from organic producers. By choosing organic products, you'll also avoid exposure to bovine growth hormone and antibiotic residues. And avoid low- or reduced-fat products; opt for full-fat whenever possible.

CHOOSE ORGANIC VEGETABLES AND FRUITS. Whenever available and budget permits, make organic your first choice, especially when the exterior of the food is consumed, as with blueberries and broccoli, for example. This helps minimize the now ubiquitous exposure we all have to pesticides, herbicides, and even genetically modified foods, and reduces the potential to be exposed to their endocrine-disruptive, cancer-causing, weight-loss-blocking effects. If you cannot choose organic, at the very least rinse fruits and veggies thoroughly in warm water to minimize pesticide and herbicide residues.

DON'T OVERLY RESTRICT SALT. For most of us engaging in a grain-free lifestyle, light to moderate use of mineral-rich forms of salt, such as sea salt, is actually healthier than severely restricting salt, particularly when that salt is combined with healthy foods rich in potassium (such as from vegetables, avocados, or coconut). In fact, advice to severely restrict salt has been formally retracted in view of clinical studies that demonstrate increased cardiovascular death with salt restriction of 1,500 mg per day or less. Average salt intake in the United States is 3,400 mg, which may be a perfectly fine level in a grain-free lifestyle.

There can be problems, however, with unlimited salt use, as salt intakes of 6,000 to 10,000 mg per day can indeed be associated with adverse cardiovascular effects. If you have kidney disease, edema, or severe hypertension, you may develop salt sensitivity and should adhere to the sodium prescription provided by your doctor.

BE CAREFUL OF PRESCRIPTION DRUGS AND NUTRITIONAL SUPPLEMENTS. Examine any nutritional supplements, protein powders, and prescription drugs for wheat- or other grain-related ingredients. For nutritional supplements, consult the ingredient list. If there is something suspicious, such as "hydrolyzed vegetable protein," consider finding a replacement product. While we are careful how we use the gluten-free concept, this is an area where a gluten-free claim can be helpful. For resources to help determine if your prescription drug contains a problem ingredient, see Appendix B.

SURVIVE THE DISASTER

Imagine you and your family endure a hurricane that ripped through your home, tearing shingles from the roof, blasting through windows, and uprooting trees. Everyone in the house is shaken but alive. Neighbors and friends are no better off, all having to pull themselves out of the rubble.

That may be where you're starting in your Wheat Belly 10-Day Detox: addled, disoriented, and confused as to why all your best dietary and exercise efforts went unrewarded. Now it's time to rebuild. You won't, of course, have to replant trees or replace windows, but you will have to declare a health state-of-emergency and acquire new nutritional tools and rethink your approach to food, weight, and health to rebuild from this health disaster called grains.

The first three steps discussed in this chapter will get you started, bulldozing your way to a new lifestyle. Now let's get some new paint and furniture in that house and make it pretty and livable again.

CHAPTER 3

OVERCOME THE ADDICTION

Successfully Surviving Detoxification and Withdrawal

WHILE I'D PREFER to talk about all the wonderful successes you can enjoy by following this new lifestyle, we have to take a few moments to talk about some things that seem more like sordid scenes from *Traffic* or *Scarface*. There are no grimy inner-city drug houses here or surreptitious cash exchanges, but there are going to be some murky, disagreeable days ahead that you need to know how to deal with if you are going to enjoy success with the Wheat Belly 10-Day Detox. The heightened drama of the next several days may match that of the latest episode of *The Young and the Restless* with the same level of tantrums and hysterics, but without the backstabbing and secret romances. You may even shed some tears through the process, but everyone survives.

Stop eating broccoli or walnuts, and there is no detoxification or withdrawal process. Stop eating beef or pork, and there is no nausea, sleep disruption, diarrhea, or headache. Stop eating wheat and grains . . . and all hell can break loose emotionally and physically, even making you question whether this process is really healthy. This is all part of the reprogramming of your body, an unavoidable process that precedes all the wonderful changes that will unfold.

Don't be fooled. Recall that the gliadin protein of wheat and related proteins in other grains (secalin in rye, hordein in barley, zein in corn—the four worst) yield opiates that bind to the brain and cause addictive eating behavior, cravings, and constant hunger. Once you stop this source of opiates—grains—there is a clear-cut opiate withdrawal syndrome that may dominate the first few days of your detoxification process.

JULIE, 51, artist, Wisconsin

"Day 1 was good until I hit a wall after dinner. The next 36 hours were short of hell. Really fatigued, then angry and anxious, too. My muscles and joints ached so bad, it was hard to stand up. The worst of the emotional distress and aches went away after the first 48 hours. I began feeling much better Day 5 and forward. My hot flashes were terrible the first 2 nights. They are better now."

ESCAPE THE DARK DIETARY CORNERS OF GRAINS

Someone addicted to heroin, morphine, or Oxycontin will, when their supply of drugs dries up, experience anxiety, nausea, sweating, dysphoria (dark moods), muscle aches, abdominal cramps, vomiting, diarrhea, and headache, a withdrawal process necessary to detoxify from the effects of opiate addiction. It is a predictable and painful process, not uncommonly bad enough to be undertaken in a hospital. Bid farewell to your last bit of wheat, rye, barley, and corn, and you can experience anxiety, nausea, sweating, dysphoria, muscle aches, abdominal cramps, vomiting, diarrhea, incapacitating fatigue, and headache—an opiate withdrawal process necessary to detoxify from the effects of grains. It won't be bad enough to require hospitalization, but it can still be pretty awful.

Not everyone experiences withdrawal, but those who do describe an unpleasant experience that disrupts lives, annoys family and friends, impairs school and work performance, and causes you to miss yoga class or poker night. (Interestingly, *all* of our detox panelists experienced some form of withdrawal, ranging from mild to pretty nasty.)

Some people with chronic joint pain or migraine headaches will experience a worsening of their symptoms during this withdrawal period, part of the impaired pain tolerance that is characteristic of opiate withdrawal. It does not mean that your condition is getting worse; it means that your tolerance to the pain is temporarily reduced. Do what you must during this period to get through, such as taking the drugs you've been prescribed for migraine headaches. But know that this will be short-lived.

Typically, the withdrawal process lasts for about 5 days, though it can last as briefly as a day or as long as several weeks (thankfully uncommon). If I had my way, I would spare you this process, but it is a necessary, unavoidable rite of passage that you must endure to get to the other side.

Don't fall into the trap of believing that this early experience, because it can be so unpleasant, must therefore be bad for health. It is not. It is a form of detoxification, a withdrawal syndrome, a crucial process to undo the effects of addiction. Just as an alcoholic who wishes to rid her life of alcohol can only do so by stopping the bourbon and whiskey and suffering the withdrawal consequences, so the detoxification from grain-derived opiates must be endured to overcome the addictive, appetite-stimulating effects and declare your freedom from its physical, mental, and emotional grip.

If you thought you were just going to do this detox thing to lose a few pounds, you are now beginning to appreciate that there are many more dimensions to wheat and grain consumption than just weight. We're talking about having to endure processes you thought didn't apply to you, opiate addictions that even involve children, allowing a form of coercive behavior manipulation that was, and still is, widely exploited by food manufacturers (partially explaining, for instance, why wheat and grains are present in virtually every processed food). But understand this basic principle, and you are on track to be freed of these effects and achieve a level of freedom of appetite, impulse control, health, and weight that you have likely never before experienced. You will be liberated.

Just as an alcoholic can temporarily halt the tremors, paranoia, and hallucinations of alcohol withdrawal with a calming shot (or 10) of whiskey, so can you turn off the uncomfortable process of grain withdrawal by consuming any wheat, rye, barley, or corn product. But you'll also halt your return to health, and you'll have to start the process all over again, suffering all the same symptoms, if you have any hopes of conquering this demon. Even small, inadvertent exposures to grain ingredients, in, say, a package of instant soup mix or a granola bar, are enough to halt the detoxification/withdrawal process. Follow the guidelines we discussed in Chapter 2 to effectively protect yourself from such exposures and avoid prolonging the agony.

So, if you are going to have grain opiate withdrawal, you are going to have grain opiate withdrawal. There is just no way around it. Thankfully, however, the process can be partially softened by a number of strategies that we discuss next.

GRAIN WITHDRAWAL: SMOOTHING THE TRANSITION

You are facing the prospect of withdrawal, a tumultuous physical and emotional storm. This can be terrifying, especially now that you know it can involve fatigue, nausea, anxiety, headache, lightheadedness, leg cramps, and depression, as well as powerful cravings for the foods you are avoiding. Many people have previously experienced a small taste of this syndrome with brief lapses in grain intake, though they probably didn't recognize it as grain withdrawal. They might have dismissed the anxiety and headache, for instance, as the effects of hunger or physical weakness which were promptly relieved with a few pretzels or bites of leftover pizza. But with the complete removal of grains from your diet, those feelings are going to persist for a while.

Is there an emotional electroshock therapy that might zap you out of this experience, an antidote to the rigors of removing this mind-active drug, a laxative that purges the poison, anything you can do to smooth the grain withdrawal syndrome? Yes, there are steps you can take to make it less nasty. Nothing will completely ablate the experience, no general anesthetic to make it painless, but you can take measures to soften the blow. Here are a few strategies.

Choose a Nonstressful Period to Experience Withdrawal

If you have the luxury of managing your time, choose a period when you don't anticipate high stress or extended travel. Don't choose, for instance, the week you expect to start a new and challenging work project, or when a disruptive mother-in-law who criticizes your every move is planning to visit, or the week before your dissertation is due, or the week you are planning to fly to Europe. Ideally, choose a long weekend or period of several days without such obligations. And you should pamper yourself: Watch funny movies and laugh (surely you could watch *Bridesmaids* again), enjoy a glass of wine (but just one—any more and your ability to start the weight-loss process will be turned off), lie in the sun, get a massage. Like a bad hangover, this will pass.

But be certain to not use this as an excuse to procrastinate. You should have a very good reason to delay the process, such as those listed above, but don't avoid starting just because you might be stressed or inconvenienced. To be freed of all these awful effects, you have to start sometime, sooner rather than later.

Don't Exercise

That may sound odd, given the benefits of exercise. But exercising during the withdrawal process is like trying to jog, swim, or jump rope while suffering the flu: It will be a miserable experience minus the sinus congestion. Don't torture yourself, and don't feel guilty for not exercising. At most, do something at a leisurely pace: Go for a walk in the woods or around your neighborhood, or take a casual bike ride. But it would be counterproductive to force yourself to run, bike hard, or strength-train, as the effort will make you feel worse. Rest assured that, once the fireworks of withdrawal are over, you will feel so wonderful that physical activities and exercise will not just be possible again without all the discomfort, but you will feel eager for the freedom and movement of vigorous physical activity.

Hydrate

The physiologic changes experienced during this process, such as a precipitous drop in insulin, also reverse the sodium retention of wheat and grain consumption, causing fluid loss (diuresis) and reduction in inflammation. If you don't compensate by hydrating more than usual over the first few days, light-headedness, nausea, and leg cramps can result. Hydration is therefore crucial during this first week.

A great habit to start the day right is to drink a pint of (filtered, nonchlorinated, nonfluoridated) water immediately upon awakening, since we wake up dehydrated after lying flat and mouth breathing during sleep through the night. You can recognize proper hydration if your urine is nearly clear, not a dark, concentrated yellow. The best liquid to hydrate with is water. Drink it plain or with a twist of lemon, lime, or a few drops of flavored stevia. Also, see the Coconut Electrolyte Replacement Water rec- ipe on page 152.

If you are taking a prescription diuretic for high blood pres- sure, such as hydrochlorothiazide or chlorthalidone, speak to the prescribing doctor about the possibility of stopping it during your withdrawal process and onward, as diuretics force you to be dehydrated to do their work, which is obviously counterproduc- tive (not to mention diuretics deplete potassium and magnesium, raise blood sugar, and barely work anyway).

YVETTE, 50, history professor, New Jersey

"Headache was the biggest symptom for me. I think that Day 9 was actu- ally the first day I did not wake up with a headache or have one throughout the day. I had some hunger here and there. I also had some loose bowel movements that cleared up pretty quickly. I was more tired than usual. On one of the days, I felt very discouraged because I didn't seem to be losing any weight and I also felt especially clumsy that day. I bumped into things and just felt generally miserable, but it passed in a day or so.

"I took ibuprofen a few times and napped when I could. I also had a massage one day and went for a swim. Frankly, none of the withdrawal was so bad. It was more of a nagging discomfort most of the time. So, naps, ibuprofen, and Peanut Butter Cup Fat Blasters (page 142) were my go-to withdrawal helpers."

Use Some Salt

Sprinkle sea salt or other mineral-containing salt on your food to compensate for the loss of urinary salt that develops due to drop- ping insulin levels. Salt, along with hydration, addresses the light-headedness and leg cramps that commonly occur during withdrawal. (Factor in a sodium restriction if you have kidney disease or other reason to limit salt, however.)

Strict limitation on salt use is another widely held notion that, along with limiting fat and eating grains, dissolves with the health transformations of wheat and grain elimination. Have some salt: You will feel better if you do. (If you use iodized salt, it is still worth supplementing iodine as a nutritional supplement, as discussed in Chapter 4, since iodized salt is a fairly unreliable source of iodine, particularly if the salt canister sits for more than a few weeks, since iodine evaporates quite quickly.)

Get Over Your Fat Phobia and Eat Fat

It's built right into the three steps of the detox, but despite that, many people really struggle with following through on this strategy and shutting out the crippling dietary advice of the last 30 years. To make matters worse, the world of food has so deeply taken "cut your fat and cholesterol" to heart that it is often difficult to find, for instance, full-fat dairy products or be served a fatty cut of meat at a restaurant.

If you are hungry or experience cravings during your detox, it nearly always reflects failure to take in sufficient fat. While this can also reflect the withdrawal process from grain-derived opiates, it can be compounded by the failure to take in enough fat.

You may shock your family and friends as you proceed to not trim the fat off your meats, or eat a big hunk of full-fat cheese, or prepare your eggs swimming in bacon grease, but you're not doing this for their approval. You are doing it for health. You might consider carrying some Fat Blasters (see recipes in Chapter 6) around with you in a sealable, water- and oil-tight container (in case the oil melts) to consume when hunger or cravings strike.

Supplement Magnesium

Magnesium deficiency is widespread and is associated over time with osteoporosis, hypertension, higher blood sugar, muscle cramps, and heart rhythm disorders. Magnesium deficiency is common and can magnify some of the symptoms of withdrawal from grains, particularly leg cramps and sleep disruption.

Magnesium supplementation can therefore have dramatic benefits during withdrawal. Unfortunately, most magnesium supplements are better laxatives than sources of absorbable magnesium, responsible for loose stools without relief from any of the health issues. Among the best absorbed with the least laxative effect is magnesium malate at a dose of 1,200 mg two or three times per day (weight of the magnesium + malate, not just "elemental" magnesium, i.e., the magnesium by itself; this provides 180 mg elemental magnesium per 1,200 mg tablet or capsule, or 360 mg per day).

Another way to get supplemental magnesium is to make your own inexpensive and wonderfully effective magnesium bicarbonate, the most absorbable form of all, if you don't mind a bit of effort. Because it is very hygroscopic (water absorbent), no manufacturer sells magnesium bicarbonate in dry form, so you have to make it yourself. The formula for Coconut Magnesium Water can be found on page 150.

While we are introducing magnesium supplementation to smooth the grain withdrawal process, it is something you should consider continuing for the long term, well after the withdrawal process subsides.

Supplement Tryptophan or 5-Hydroxytryptophan

Brain serotonin levels can drop with weight loss, resulting in food cravings, low mood, irritability, anger, and argumentativeness. While the conventional medical answer is to prescribe brain serotonin–increasing antidepressant drugs, you can increase serotonin levels a natural way and reduce the negative emotions and cravings of the withdrawal process. Some people like the effects of these supplements so much, especially the favorable effects on mood, that they continue taking them long after the wheat and grain withdrawal is nothing more than a bad memory.

Brain serotonin levels can be increased by taking the nutritional supplements tryptophan or its closely related 5-hydroxytryptophan (5-HTP). These supplements have proven effective in clinical trials where they have been used to combat depression and even alcohol withdrawal, resulting in improved mood (helping people become less argumentative and less aggressive), fewer negative thoughts, and reduced carbohydrate cravings.

Tryptophan can be taken during the day, e.g., 500 to 1,000 mg three times per day. Alternatively, it can be taken at a higher dose once per day at bedtime to encourage sleep at a dose of 1,000 to 3,000 mg. Tryptophan is most effective taken on an empty stomach.

If tryptophan is not available to you, the more widely available 5-HTP, taken at a dose of 50 to 100 mg three times per day, exerts similar effect. Or, as with tryptophan, a single daily bedtime dose of 100 to 300 mg can be used to improve sleep and obtain the daytime benefits.

BREAKTHROUGH

You may remember your personal experience of detoxification from "healthy whole grains" as among the more awful things you've had to endure in your lifetime, alongside quitting cigarette smoking or being audited by the taxman. You now know that grain detox is not about a sorrowful break with nostalgia, just cutting carbs, or denying yourself calories. It is about breaking the physiologic addiction of dietary opiates, shaking off the hold they had over you and your behavior and health, and detoxifying from their effects.

Emerge on the other side, however, whether it required a few days or a few weeks, and you encounter a brighter, happier side of life that you may have thought you'd lost. It starts your journey back to health, as well, as the pounds fall off, visceral fat mobilizes, the gastrointestinal tract heals, skin clears, and retained water is released, while your mind becomes clearer, appetite shrinks, sleep becomes deeper and restorative, and daytime energy soars. It is truly like a glorious rainbow after a dark storm, a genuine breakthrough for a new future.

The opiate withdrawal process that occurs with ceasing all wheat and grains was something you had little control over, having to endure it whether you liked it or not. But, after this period of helplessness, you are now in wonderfully complete control over appetite, weight, and health. That, perhaps, is among the most satisfying aspects of this lifestyle: No longer are you controlled by food, food manufacturers, or marketing. This lifestyle puts *you* back in control.

But you're not finished. Removing a dietary toxin and reorganizing your daily meal routine are your big first steps. Next we'll discuss the additional steps required to reverse all the adverse health consequences that, although initially caused by wheat and grains, can persist even in their absence. Recognize and then correct these additional factors, and you will take health, weight, and appearance to even higher levels.

CHAPTER 4

A SUCKER PUNCH
TO THE WHEAT BELLY

WE'VE TALKED ABOUT the full frontal assault that you are going to launch on health and weight with the three starting steps of your Wheat Belly 10-Day Detox. Let's now land a blow that knocks the wind out of all remaining barriers to ideal health and weight with a sucker punch to their softer parts.

You now hopefully understand why 100 percent elimination—not 90 percent reduction, not 6 days out of 7, not every day except holidays, but total elimination, down to the very last bread crumb—of wheat and grains packs such a powerful punch in launching your detox process. And you now understand why it is the unavoidable and absolutely necessary initial step before the rest of your detox program can unfold properly and naturally, allowing a virtual reprogramming of your body's physiology.

Let's talk about some simple nutritional methods that accelerate your progress, restore health even further, support your body's healing, and will build up momentum that continues well beyond the initial 10 days. We are going to address the crucial health-restoring issues of bowel flora, the status of vitamin D and other nutrients, iodine and thyroid health, and the role of fiber.

SMASH THROUGH
YOUR HEALING CEILING

With grains, the cause of all your problems, now removed, healing can finally proceed. But because your body has taken a beating at so many levels—gastrointestinal, metabolic, joints, immune system, and others—from years of grain consumption, removing them does not fully reverse every abnormal situation they created. There's more to do to ensure recovery. Failing to take these additional steps will deprive you of the full benefit of the detoxification process, and you will hit a healing ceiling. You must therefore find ways to incorporate these strategies to ensure that you take health and weight all the way through to your goals.

It's not very different than recovering from alcoholism. If an alcoholic takes her last swig of whiskey on Tuesday, will she be back in perfect health by Wednesday? Thursday? Next week? Obviously, no. Beyond the first week or so of alcohol detoxification and withdrawal, she has plenty of healing to do: recovery of her liver, heart, brain, and gastrointestinal system—just about every organ damaged by the toxic effects of excessive, daily alcohol coupled with the nutritional deficiencies of a neglectful diet.

The dramatic lifestyle shift of wheat and grain elimination will take you through similar changes. You may have to endure the emotional and physical uproar of grain-induced opiate withdrawal and start feeling tons better, but health will not be fully restored until additional efforts are undertaken. These efforts are not required because removing grains leaves you lacking something; they are necessary because you need to undo all unhealthy effects caused by grains that can persist even in their absence. But your detox process will proceed faster, be more complete, and bring you closer to ideal health, upping the chances that you will also look the picture of perfect health.

Let's focus on the issues that emerge front and center in this 10-day detox period that must be managed for you to experience full and enduring success.

MANAGE YOUR GARDEN OF BOWEL FLORA

From consuming grains as well as sugary foods and soft drinks for years, eating meats laced with antibiotic residues, being exposed to genetically modified foods containing built-in pesticides, and taking intermittent prescription antibiotics or acid reflux drugs to drinking chlorinated tap water and aspartame in diet soda and ingesting emulsifying agents in processed foods—people today have managed to utterly discombobulate the composition of microorganisms inhabiting their intestines. These organisms, however, are not only important for bowel health but also critical for overall health. Having a healthy, diverse profile of microorganisms in your intestines helps control weight, improves metabolic factors (reduced triglycerides, blood sugars, and insulin), reduces blood pressure, encourages bowel regularity, prevents colon cancer, and even influences sleep quality and mental health. When you remove grains, a major factor disrupting bowel flora has been removed. This represents a wonderful time to reestablish bowel flora that facilitates health and brings you closer to achieving your goals.

It helps to view bowel flora as being like a backyard garden. In springtime, you prepare the soil and plant seeds. Can you then walk away and come back in 2 months and have a successful garden bursting with courgettes and squash? Of course not. You should have also watered, fertilized, and weeded your garden with some frequency. This is how it works with bowel flora: We need to plant "seeds" (probiotics that contain organisms you may lack), then "water and fertilize" the garden (prebiotic fibers or resistant starches that nourish the preferred species that yield benefits to the host, i.e., you). Both probiotics and prebiotics are essential components of this process.

We start by "seeding" your intestines with a high-potency probiotic supplement. We need to ensure that there are adequate numbers of organisms to make a difference. This generally means a "colony-forming unit," or CFU, count of at least 30 billion to 50 billion per day, taken in capsule form. It also means providing a wide diversity of species. The best probiotics typically contain a dozen or more species, such as *Lactobacillus plantarum* and *Bifidobacterium infantis*. But, just as you do not need to plant seeds every day of the growing season to have a successful garden, so you do not need to supplement probiotics every day for the rest of your life. You only need to take them for a limited time, e.g., 6 to 8 weeks, long enough to reseed your intestines with healthy species—provided you properly nourish them. This strategy will therefore outlast your initial 10-day detox, but it stacks the odds in favor of a successful bowel flora transition.

The "water and fertilizer" for your bowel flora come from some unusual sources, since we are trying to choose modern equivalents of primitive sources. These are fibers or starches that are indigestible by our own digestive apparatus (and thereby do not raise blood sugar) but are digestible by micro-organisms in the bowels. These fibers are distinct, however, from cellulose—wood fiber—the fiber in bran cereals and other products that provide "bulk," or indigestible filler, and yield bowel regularity. We want more than bulk and bowel regularity. We want facilitation of weight loss, improved metabolic measures, better sleep, etc., that comes from the unique form of fibers that are metabolized by bowel flora to fatty acids and yield these wonderful health benefits. We obtain such fibers from:

Green bananas (truly green and unripe) and plantains:
Up to 27 g fiber in one medium banana

Raw white potato (peeled): 20 g fiber per 1 medium
(3½ inches long)

Hummus or roasted chickpeas: 15 g fiber per 55 g (2 oz)
(10 g net carbohydrates)

Inulin powder: 5 g fiber per teaspoon

Fructooligosaccharide (FOS) powder: 5 g fiber per
teaspoon

Lentils: 2.5 g fiber in 95 g (3½ oz) cup (11 g net
carbohydrates)

Beans: 1.8 g fiber in 50 g (2 oz) (11 g net carbohydrates)

We aim for a total prebiotic fiber intake of 20 g per day. The easiest way to accomplish this is to include a coarsely chopped green banana or raw white potato in a smoothie every day. Wheat Belly Detox Shake recipes (see Chapter 5) in the 10-Day Menu Plan incorporate the needed quantities of these fibers. Once you've graduated from your 10-day initiation, you can obtain your fibers by other means than the shakes. Inulin or fructooligosaccharide (FOS) powders, found in health food stores, are an especially convenient way to obtain such fibers. In addition to the convenience of inulin and FOS powders, there are some other convenient commercial products that can be used, listed in Appendix B.

I like to slice or chop a raw potato to include in salads, blend a chopped raw potato or green banana into a smoothie, add a couple of teaspoons of powdered inulin to various dishes, and dip vegetables or grain-free crackers into hummus. Consuming small quantities—e.g., no more than ¼ of a tea cup per meal—of lentils, chickpeas, and starchy beans (black, kidney, white, lima) adds to your daily total. Root vegetables (onions, sweet potatoes, parsnips, swede, maca, celeriac, daikon, and others) likewise add a gram or two of these fibers, but be careful to not exceed your

15 g net carbs per meal, most important during your initial 10-day detox experience and during any weight-loss effort.

You can get creative with ways to include prebiotic fibers in your daily routine, even slipping them into your family's diet. For example, slice a green banana into 1-inch pieces and dip the slices into one bar of melted 85 percent cocoa dark chocolate. (Use waxed paper to keep the chocolate from sticking to the plate and store in the refrigerator to keep the banana from ripening; they're good for about 3 days.) These chocolate-covered banana bites provide 3 to 4 g prebiotic fibers per bite. Add inulin or FOS fibers to dishes such as Apricot Ginger "Granola" (page 108). Or, for the kids, pour a glass of coconut milk and add unsweetened cocoa powder, a few drops of liquid stevia, and 1 teaspoon inulin or FOS. As you get comfortable with the sources of these fibers and begin to appreciate the power of this bowel flora-supporting strategy, you will see that there are many opportunities throughout the day to supplement your intake.

An important precaution: Start slowly at no more than 10 g prebiotic fibers. Only use, for instance, about half of the green banana or half of the raw potato in your smoothie to start, and build up over the 10-day detox period, or else abdominal discomfort and excessive gas can result. You also want to allow the probiotic supplement to provide the healthy bacterial species that you are trying to grow to take "root" before you begin adding the prebiotic fibers. (These limitations are built into the 10-Day Menu Plan to make it easy for you.) The benefits of this powerful strategy, such as lower blood pressure and deeper sleep, develop slowly over 2 to 3 months and longer as healthy species proliferate and exert their metabolic benefits. The key is long-term consistency while varying your choice of these fibers from day to day to encourage diversity of species. These are habits you want to continue for the rest of your life.

RUN NAKED IN A TROPICAL SUN ... OR SUPPLEMENT VITAMIN D

Restoration of vitamin D, in my view, is second only to wheat and grain elimination as the most powerful tool for health available. Even after 10 years of having my patients supplement vitamin D to achieve healthy blood levels, I still marvel at the wonderful effects that develop. Although vitamin D absorption from the small quantities in food is impaired only in people with celiac disease, Crohn's disease, and some other intestinal conditions, it is so important to your overall health that I place it front and center in your Wheat Belly 10-Day Detox program. It plays so many crucial roles in health that doctors should be experts in vitamin D, but that is sadly not generally the case. Doctors and other health care professionals are experts at dispensing drugs and procedures, not health. So vitamin D, as critical as it is for health, is generally left to you to manage properly. But you can do an expert job for you and your family.

Humans were meant to obtain vitamin D from sun exposure over large surface areas of skin, supplemented by the modest quantities provided by seafood, shellfish, organs of land animals (especially liver), egg yolks, and mushrooms. But in modern life, many of us live in colder climates, wear clothes much of the year, stay indoors year-round, and (wrongly) avoid foods like egg yolks and liver while only occasionally eating seafood. We also lose much of the ability to activate vitamin D in our skin as we get older; by age 40, most people have lost a major part of this ability and fail to achieve optimal levels even with a dark Caribbean tan.

Restore vitamin D to healthy levels and wonderful things happen: improved mood, clearer thinking, better bone health and protection from osteoporosis, reduced blood sugar and blood pressure, and improved physical performance and protection from dementia and cancer—compounding many of the wonderful effects begun by wheat and grain elimination. Many people actually feel the beneficial effects of vitamin D restoration, especially improved mood and mental clarity, as well as relief from seasonal "blues." Inflammation and autoimmune conditions, such as rheumatoid arthritis and psoriasis, are especially responsive: The initial trigger for these conditions—wheat and grains—has been removed, but restoring vitamin D further reverses the abnormal inflammatory and immune responses that allowed these diseases to manifest.

Young people who possess the ability to activate vitamin D in the skin and enjoy plentiful sun exposure naturally develop 25-hydroxy vitamin D blood levels (the lab test that reflects vitamin D status) of 70 to 84 ng/mL or higher without adverse effect, suggesting that we can safely do likewise. I therefore advise people to take 4,000 to 8,000 international units (IUs) per day of oil-based vitamin D_3, or cholecalciferol, in gelcaps or drops, for assured absorption. This dose is sufficient to achieve a 25-hydroxy vitamin D blood level of 60 to 70 ng/mL after 2 to 3 months of supplementation in the majority of people, just like a young lifeguard with a tan. Not restricting foods such as egg yolks and liver also makes a modest contribution. Avoid vitamin D in tablet form, as it is erratically or poorly absorbed. Also avoid the D_2, or ergocalciferol, form (which is present in prescription vitamin D) as it is nonhuman and not as effective as the human form, D_3.

Because there can be wide individual variation in vitamin D intake required to achieve the same target levels in the body, it helps to obtain an occasional blood test for 25-hydroxy vitamin D that reflects your vitamin D status. Ideally, blood levels should be assessed no sooner than 3 months after initiating supplementation (since it takes that long to plateau), then reassessed every year or so to ensure that you remain within the target range.

CORRECT THE MAGNESIUM DEFICIENCY OF GRAINS

Recall that the phytates of wheat and grains block absorption of nutrients, mostly minerals. Magnesium is among those blocked, with absorption reduced by 60 percent in the presence of grains. Magnesium deficiency is further compounded by the reduced magnesium content of modern crops, our reliance on home or municipal water filtration that removes all magnesium, and the widespread use of drugs for acid reflux and ulcers that reduce magnesium absorption. Add it all up, and magnesium deficiency is the rule at the start of your program.

The American Recommended Dietary Allowance (RDA) of "elemental" magnesium (i.e., magnesium by itself) is 320 mg per day for adult females and 420 mg per day for adult males. Most people obtain around 245 mg per day—well below the RDA—while not even factoring in the impaired absorption caused by grains or drugs. Most of us therefore take in far less magnesium than we should. Because magnesium provides structural integrity to bone tissue, lack of magnesium contributes to osteoporosis. Deficiency is also associated with hypertension, higher blood sugars, muscle cramps, migraines, and heart rhythm disorders. Magnesium deficiency can express itself to an exaggerated degree during the wheat and grain withdrawal process, experienced as leg cramps and disruption of sleep in the first few days, so everyone ideally begins magnesium supplementation on Day 1 of the Wheat Belly 10-Day Detox.

We've got to be choosy with magnesium supplements, however, as most are better laxatives than forms of absorbable magnesium. Among the best absorbed tablet or capsule forms is magnesium malate at a dose of 1,200 mg two or three times per day; this provides 180 mg elemental magnesium per 1,200 mg tablet or capsule. Another better absorbed form is magnesium glycinate, 400 mg two or three times per day. If you desire looser bowel movements, then magnesium citrate, 400 mg two or three times per day, provokes a modest osmotic effect (pulling water into the colon). You will also find a simple recipe for Coconut Magnesium Water (page 150), a method of making magnesium bicarbonate, the best form of magnesium available with less potential for loose stools. (Don't do both magnesium supplements and magnesium water; take one or the other.)

It can help to increase your intake of magnesium-rich foods, as well, such as pumpkin seeds, sesame seeds, and sunflower seeds; nuts such as almonds and pecans, as well as peanuts and (unsweetened) peanut butter; and lots of spinach and other green leafy vegetables. Our Wheat Belly Detox Shakes in Chapter 5 include (optional) pumpkin seeds to substantially up your daily magnesium intake. Given the difficulties with continuing to maintain a healthy magnesium intake, supplementation and including magnesium-rich foods are habits to continue for a lifetime. (Anyone with kidney disease should not take magnesium except under supervision, as magnesium can accumulate with impaired kidney function.) Maintaining a long-term program of magnesium restoration can be an important part of your overall effort to reestablish multiple facets of grain-free health.

OMEGA-3 FATTY ACIDS MAKE WEIGHT LOSS SAFER

Omega-3 fatty acids are important during your 10-day detox. Once grains are removed from the diet, weight loss proceeds at a rapid pace for most people, a process that involves mobilization of fatty acids into the bloodstream. If a cholesterol panel were checked during active weight loss (which you should generally not have checked to avoid confusion, including the perplexed look of your doctor, eager to whip out the prescription pad), you would see high triglyceride levels, since triglycerides transport fatty acids—a natural part of the fat mobilization process of weight loss. The omega-3 fatty acids from fish oil accelerate clearance of fatty acids from the bloodstream and keep levels lower. Subduing rises in fatty acids and triglycerides makes the process of weight loss safer and helps minimize transient rises in blood pressure and blood sugar that can develop.

Infrequent consumption of seafood, aversion to organ meats, and overreliance on processed omega-6 oils in modern foods have led to deficient levels of omega-3 fatty acids in the majority of people at the start of the detox. Now that the absorption-blocking, inflammatory grains have been removed, omega-3 fatty acid absorption may improve, but intake typically remains low for most people and supplementation is necessary to achieve healthy blood levels (for everyone except the most enthusiastic fish-consuming individuals).

There are plenty of other reasons to supplement omega-3 fatty acids beyond the initial detox experience. There are, for instance, an abundance of clinical studies that demonstrate that omega-3 fatty acids, as eicosapentaenoic acid (EPA) and docosa-hexaenoic acid (DHA) obtained from fish and fish oil, yield reductions in sudden cardiac death, heart attack, heart rhythm disorders, autoimmune inflammatory conditions (especially rheumatoid arthritis and lupus), and a variety of cancers. While linolenic acid—found in flaxseeds, chia seeds, walnuts, and other sources—is biochemically an omega-3 fatty acid and is, for other reasons, a truly healthy oil, it does not yield the same benefits provided by EPA and DHA from fish and fish oil. Krill oil is likewise not a useful source of EPA and DHA, as the quantities contained are too small to make a difference, despite the over-the-top misleading marketing claims made by some manufacturers.

I advocate an intake of 3,000 to 3,600 mg per day (the dose of combined EPA and DHA, not the total weight of fish oil), divided into two doses taken before breakfast and before or after dinner. This quantity yields an ideal level of omega-3 fatty acids in the bloodstream, subdues the flood of fatty acids, provides maximal protection from cardiovascular disease, and yields anti-inflammatory benefits.

IODINE: FORGOTTEN BUT VITAL TRACE NUTRIENT FOR THYROID HEALTH

While we cannot blame grains for messing with our iodine status, deficiency is so common and can be such a stumbling block in health that it is worth knowing about. Failure to correct iodine deficiency can substantially impair your ability to lose weight, while adding to cardiovascular risk, hypertension, risk for breast conditions like fibrocystic breast disease, and water retention.

Most people have forgotten that, up until the first half of the 20th century, disfiguring goiters occurred in 20 percent of the population: large bulging thyroid glands on the front of the neck due to lack of iodine. This was an especially serious problem for people living inland, away from ocean sources of iodine. The connection between goiters and iodine deficiency led to the introduction of iodized salt in the U.S. in 1924, and the FDA urged the public to use more salt. Unfortunately, excessive salt consumption caused health problems in some susceptible individuals, prompting new advice: Reduce salt and sodium consumption. Now, in the 21st century, health-conscious people avoid iodized table salt. Others have turned to alternative sources, such as sea salt (very little iodine content), kosher salt (no iodine), and potassium chloride–based salt substitutes (no iodine). As a result, iodine deficiency and goiters are making a vigorous (and often unnoticed) comeback.

Iodine is an essential trace mineral for health. Because salivary glands and breast tissue concentrate iodine, it is required for oral health and protection from conditions such as fibrocystic breast disease. Iodine is essential for normal thyroid function, in particular, since thyroid hormones, T4 and T3, are composed of iodine (the "4" and "3" referring to the number of iodine molecules). Iodine deficiency over time leads to a thyroid gland that enlarges—a goiter, seen as a bulge on the front of the neck. However, it is not necessary to have a goiter for thyroid dysfunction to be present.

If you are marginally iodine deficient at the start of your Wheat Belly 10-Day Detox, your ability to lose weight will be impaired and benefits such as reduction in triglycerides, lower blood pressure, and improved mood will be blocked. Simply meeting the RDA of 150 mcg per day of iodine will prevent a goiter from developing and maintain a normal level of thyroid hormone production for most people, though you might do better by taking higher levels, as discussed below. Athletes and those engaged in frequent heavy physical effort are at a higher risk for iodine deficiency because of iodine loss through perspiration. Vegetarians who avoid seafood and iodized salt also have a greater likelihood of iodine deficiency than omnivores.

Relying on iodized salt is not the best method for obtaining iodine because it's difficult to know precisely how much iodine you're getting when sprinkling salt over food. The iodine content of iodized salt is also inconsistent, evaporating from the container within 4 weeks of opening. (A canister of iodized salt that's been sitting in your cupboard for, say, 6 months contains little to no iodine.) Many multivitamins or multiminerals contain the RDA for iodine. If there is any indication of hypothyroidism—such as inappropriately cold hands and feet, low energy, constipation, or thinning hair, and certainly if an enlarged thyroid is present—or you wish to supplement an iodine dose more likely to be the ideal level, then an increase in iodine to the 500 to 1,000 mcg per day range may increase thyroid hormone output if lack of iodine is the limiting factor. Iodine is readily obtained from supplements such as potassium iodide drops or kelp tablets, which are made from dried seaweed that approximates the natural, ocean-derived source. (I prefer kelp, as it provides a mixture of iodine forms.)

If symptoms of hypothyroidism are present, it is worth considering having a thyroid assessment by your health care provider. Even though wheat and grain elimination removes a common cause for autoimmune thyroid disease (especially Hashimoto's thyroiditis) that often results in hypothyroidism, thyroid tissue is fragile and usually does not recover after grains are removed. This can be identified through thyroid testing that includes measures of the thyroid hormones, free T4 and free T3 (reflecting the "free," or unbound, fractions in the bloodstream), thyroid stimulating hormone (TSH), as well as thyroid antibodies that cause inflammation and thyroid damage. Though not understood by most conventional doctors, a reverse T3 level can also be helpful, as this may reveal whether you have a blocker of the T3 thyroid hormone present that might be responsible for symptoms of hypothyroidism even when other measures are favorable. Thyroid testing can also suggest iodine deficiency with a low free T4 value (at or below the reference range), along with a slightly higher than optimal TSH of 1.5 mIU/L or greater. This is usually corrected after 3 to 6 months of iodine replacement if iodine deficiency is the cause, especially if thyroid enlargement is present.

Rarely, someone with hypothyroidism or a goiter will develop an abnormal hyperthyroid (overactive) response to iodine. This occurs because the iodine deficiency present before correction distorts thyroid function; adding iodine worsens the situation temporarily by activating hyperthyroidism, experienced as palpitations, sleeplessness, and anxiety. In this uncommon situation, iodine replacement is best undertaken several months after wheat and grain elimination has allowed thyroid inflammation to subside and with monitoring of thyroid function, as well as other assessments of thyroid status (such as thyroid ultrasound), by your health care provider. Once cleared of trouble spots such as abnormal thyroid nodules, some people succeed by increasing their dose of iodine gradually: They might start at a level below the RDA of 150 mcg per day and gradually build up by 50 to 100 mcg monthly increments over 6 months until the desired dose (e.g., 500 mcg per day) is achieved. Anyone with a history of Hashimoto's thyroiditis, Graves' disease, thyroid cancer, or thyroid nodules should supplement iodine only under the supervision of a knowledgeable health care provider.

IRON: AN IRONIC SITUATION

Some people, especially menstruating females and athletes, benefit from an assessment of iron status to stack the odds in favor of full recovery and high performance. This is particularly important if symptoms such as low energy, light-headedness, inappropriate feelings of coldness (also caused by hypothyroidism), breathlessness, or difficulty concentrating are present; these are symptoms of iron deficiency and anemia caused by iron deficiency. After blood loss, grain consumption is the second most common cause of iron deficiency anemia in the world. Recall that the phytate content of a bagel or two slices of bread is enough to reduce iron absorption by 80 to 90 percent, a situation not remedied by fortification.

Unlike our other Wheat Belly 10-Day Detox supplements, iron is one that requires a blood test before you proceed. This may not be an issue you tackle during your detox experience but something to address long term after wheat and grain removal, especially if the above symptoms were present prior to your detox and persist during and afterward. Removal of grains permits normal iron absorption to resume, and supplemental iron intake will only be necessary if low levels of the iron storage protein ferritin or if iron deficiency anemia is identified by blood tests. In these situations, several months of either over-the-counter or prescribed iron supplements may be necessary and can accelerate correction.

If iron deficiency is identified, look for iron supplements in the ferrous form: ferrous fumarate, ferrous sulfate, and ferrous gluconate. Of these, ferrous fumarate is the best absorbed (33 percent absorption) and gluconate is the least (12 percent). (There are also ferric forms that are poorly absorbed and are not recommended.) The elemental iron American RDA is 8 mg per day for males, 18 mg per day for menstruating females, and up to 27 mg per day for a pregnant mother. The various supplements should be dosed by the quantity of elemental iron, not the total weight of the tablet. Iron supplements should not be taken without a diagnosed iron deficiency, ongoing blood loss (such as through menses or pregnancy), and careful monitoring as iron overload can occur and can be toxic.

Due to inflammation of the small intestine, people diagnosed with celiac disease and Crohn's disease may require iron supplementation for longer than usual to compensate for reduced absorption. Iron deficiency, especially mild degrees as represented by low levels of ferritin but without anemia, is common in vegetarians, menstruating females, athletes, and people with hypochlorhydria (low stomach acid from prior grain consumption, diagnosed by your doctor). A ferritin level and complete blood count can determine whether these situations apply to you.

ZINC: BACK IN THE PINK

Zinc is a fascinating mineral, but one often neglected. If your goal is to recover health as quickly as possible during your detox, then addressing zinc can help. Recall that grain phytates that impair iron and magnesium absorption also impair zinc absorption, resulting in widespread deficiency among grain-consuming people. Zinc deficiency can account for symptoms such as skin

Summary: Wheat Belly Detox Supplements

Look for the supplements we use in the Wheat Belly 10-Day Detox in health food stores. Because of regional variation in brands, the reputable brands that are available to you may differ from the ones I list below. Where national brands are widely distributed, I will specify a few quality representative ones.

High-potency probiotic supplement: 30 billion to 50 billion CFUs per day for 6 to 8 weeks. My favorite brands include Garden of Life, Renew Life, and VSL#3, all of which contain a long list of preferred bacterial species, as well as high CFU counts.

Vitamin D: 4,000 to 8,000 IUs per day to start for adults, as gelcaps or drops; long-term dose adjusted to achieve a 25-hydroxy vitamin D blood level of 60 to 70 ng/mL. Excellent vitamin D preparations are widely available in many brands and surprisingly low in cost. Look for oil-based gelcaps (that look like little fish oil capsules) or liquid drops, but not tablets.

Magnesium: Preferably magnesium malate, 1,200 mg two or three times per day, or magnesium glycinate, 400 mg two or three times per day; or magnesium citrate, 400 mg two or three times per day. (If elemental magnesium—i.e., magnesium without the weight of malate, glycinate, or citrate—is specified on your supplement, aim for around 400 mg magnesium per day.) Source Naturals, NOW, and KAL are excellent brands.

Fish oil: 3,000 to 3,600 mg per day of EPA and DHA, divided into two doses. Among my preferred brands are Nordic Naturals, Ascenta Nutra-Sea, and Carlson.

Iodine: 500 to 1,000 mcg per day as potassium iodide drops or kelp tablets. Like vitamin D, there are many excellent preparations available at low cost.

Iron: Look for supplements in the ferrous form and take only if low ferritin levels or iron deficiency anemia is identified; the dose depends on the severity of anemia and the form chosen. Sundown Naturals, Feosol, and Pure Encapsulations are among preferred brands.

Zinc: 10 to 15 mg per day of (elemental) zinc as gluconate, sulfate, or acetate. Twinlab, Thorne, and NOW provide great choices.

rashes, distortions of taste perception, unexplained diarrhea, impaired growth and development in children, increased susceptibility to infection, and poor wound healing.

Zinc supplementation can be especially important during your first few grain-free months as gastrointestinal health recovers from the destruction previously wrought by grains. The American RDA of zinc for adults is 11 mg per day for males, 8 mg per day for females, 11 mg for pregnant females, and 12 mg per day for lactating females. Much of your daily zinc needs can be obtained through food. For example, 175 g (6 oz) of braising steak provides 6 mg of zinc, 2 slices of pork loin provide 5.8 mg, 110 g (4 oz) of chicken breast provides 1.0 mg, and 75 g (3 oz) of Alaskan king crab provides 6.5 mg. After the first few months, just including such foods in their diets is all that most people need to do.

A zinc supplement should be considered during the 10-day detox and continued for the first several months. Look for zinc gluconate, zinc sulfate, and zinc acetate and examine the quantity of elemental zinc in the preparation, not total weight. Because zinc supplements are indeed meant to supplement dietary intake, a modest additional intake of 10 to 15 mg of elemental zinc per day is all that is needed. Vegans and vegetarians typically require larger doses, such as 15 to 25 mg per day, since they avoid zinc-rich animal products and commonly rely on legumes that also contain phytates that block zinc absorption. Soaking legumes for several hours reduces their phytate content, a useful strategy for people with marginal zinc intakes. People who begin their grain-free journey with inflammatory bowel diseases or other malabsorptive conditions or who take thiazide diuretics (such as hydrochlorothiazide, chlorthalidone, or metolazone) almost always start with severe zinc deficiency, so higher levels of supplementation may be required. Blood zinc levels are of limited usefulness, as they underestimate tissue levels. Nonetheless, if a blood level is obtained and is below the "reference" range, or is at the lower end of that range, zinc deficiency is highly likely. Zinc supplementation of 10 to 15 mg per day in this situation is safe and effective.

DON'T SWEAT THE FIBER

People often fear that, minus grains, they will lack fiber and wage a constant battle to keep their bowels functioning and face a future of constipation, pushing, and hemorrhoids. Not true, provided you follow this smarter way of obtaining fiber, while taking measures to feed bowel flora.

Bran breakfast cereal, now out of your repertoire, is a sad excuse for achieving bowel health and belongs with laxatives and stool softeners in the trash. The belief that grains must be among our sources of fiber is a recent notion at odds with human nutritional habits from the past several million years. Fiber can be readily obtained from legumes, tubers, vegetables, fruits, nuts, and seeds, allowing for superior bowel health without constipation, hemorrhoids, or colon cancer. Healthy fiber, as well as prebiotic or resistant fibers, can be reliably obtained in adequate quantities without grains.

Much of the fiber provided by grains is of the indigestible cellulose form, the same found in wood. Cellulose and related fibers are indigestible by both humans and bowel flora, thereby passing through, yielding "bulk" that has been mistaken for bowel health. Nonetheless, plentiful beneficial cellulose-type fibers can be obtained from nuts and seeds. For example:

Almonds, ½ cup	6 g total fiber
Brazil nuts, ½ cup	5.2 g total fiber
Peanuts, ½ cup	6.2 g total fiber
Pecans, ½ cup	5.2 g total fiber
Sesame seeds, ½ cup	12.7 g total fiber
Sunflower seeds, ½ cup	6 g total fiber
Walnuts, ½ cup	3.3 g total fiber

Vegetables, mushrooms, fruit, coconut, and cocoa are other important sources of fiber, a mixture of digestible and indigestible fiber forms. Other foods that figure prominently in the Wheat Belly lifestyle are substantial sources of fiber. For example, 1 cup of cooked spinach provides 4.3 g total fiber, two stalks of broccoli provide 11.8 g, 10 spears of asparagus provide 3 g, ¼ cup coconut flour provides 9 g, one avocado provides 13.5 g, and five large strawberries provide 5 g. If ideal daily intake of fiber is estimated to be 25 to 40 g or more per day, obtaining this value is no problem if you include some nuts and seeds in your diet, coconut and cocoa, some sources of prebiotic fibers (ideally 20 g per day), and vegetables and fruits. Adding some ground golden flaxseeds or chia seeds can boost fiber intake even further: ½ cup flaxseeds adds 23 g of total fiber; ¼ cup chia seeds, 15 g fiber.

Provided your diet is rich in these foods as well as in sources of prebiotic fibers—and not in candy bars, chewing gum, and soft drinks—obtaining healthy quantities of all forms of fiber is virtually effortless, no pushing required.

A WHEAT BELLY KNOCKOUT

You are now well on your way to not just detoxifying your body from wheat and grains, but also throwing an upper cut to the chin for all the unhealthy distortions left after a lifetime of eating "healthy whole grains." Only after you've knocked out all the destructiveness of wheat and grains from your life and started the healing process from the health pummeling you've endured can you raise your arms in triumph.

In the next chapter, we get down to business and craft your new lifestyle with a fast-paced, day-by-day 10-Day Menu Plan—completely new to the Wheat Belly program—that incorporates the strategies for health we've covered so far. You and your family will be eating your way to astounding levels of health.

WHEAT BELLY 10-DAY DETOX

Eat Your Way Back to Health with This 10-Day Menu Plan

BECAUSE THE WHEAT Belly lifestyle you are about to embark upon is such a dramatic departure from prior eating habits, and because there is a good chance that you will have to endure the rigors of withdrawal for at least the first half of this process, here is a 10-Day Menu Plan complete with recipes to help guide you through, day by day, step by step, showing you how to eat your way back to health. This Menu Plan can be your beacon of light that keeps you on track while you and your family enjoy filling and delicious meals. It provides a road map for those moments when you are lost and wandering around in the darkness that can be the wheat and grain withdrawal process, guiding you back to the right path.

You won't find any odd-tasting green juices in this detoxification process, no program of repeated enemas to "cleanse" the colon, no magical properties ascribed to teas, mysterious pills, or incantations. You will find a logical, systematic, grain-free process to enjoy foods without health or weight downsides. In the interests of getting started quickly and putting the pedal to the floor to accelerate your success, I introduce this rapid-fire process exclusively here in this book; it was not provided in any previous Wheat Belly book. You will therefore find quick-to-prepare, straightforward breakfasts, lunches, dinners, and snacks that all adhere to the Wheat Belly 10-Day Detox principles discussed, all aimed at getting you detoxified from the health damage previously incurred from grains in as short a time as possible. Some of these recipes are not just recipes for healthy, tasty food, but play a crucial role in the health transformation of the detox process. I will show you how to weave in a daily Wheat Belly Detox Shake, for example, that helps your gastrointestinal tract heal by providing prebiotic fibers needed by bowel flora. I've tried to cover every eventuality—short of making the meals for you and doing the dishes.

I also wanted this menu to introduce you to some of the wonderful wheat- and grain-free dishes we enjoy while living this lifestyle to help you and your family recognize that the

---

ELAINE, 40, realtor, Connecticut

"I have noticed that since my wheat/grain elimination, my bowel movements are smoother, less straining. The first 2 days I was fatigued more than usual and had feelings of vertigo when walking, but that has subsided. I noticed that my wedding ring is a bit loose. Sleep has been wonderful, and I haven't snored, per my husband. My sinuses have always been an issue; I've always been congested. I can breathe through my nose without problems since Saturday [the start of the detox]. I am a bit on the hungry side, but instead of reaching for chips, I have a Fat Blaster or veggies. I haven't had any acid reflux or GORD issues since Saturday, which is truly amazing. Usually, I would be reaching for the Tums before bed, yet I haven't had any since the start."

Wheat Belly lifestyle does *not* involve deprivation, but is a rich, varied, and delicious way to live that even includes familiar favorites like pizza—a dish featured on Day 1 of your Menu Plan. The recipes will introduce you, for example, to wheat-free cooking and baking methods that will show you how to make fragrant flatbreads, to create rich sauces by using safe thickeners such as coconut flour, to get comfortable with the use of safe sweeteners, and to whip up dishes like "potato" salad or breakfast fry-ups without being tripped up by problem ingredients like cooked potatoes. Aside from the Wheat Belly Detox Shakes (pages 101–107), all of the recipes in the Menu Plan and in the subsequent Secret Sauce and Secret Weapons chapters are appropriate for the rest of the family. You can therefore make these dishes for you to enjoy on your own, or you can share them with everyone else.

Wheat Belly Detox Shakes begin on Day 3. The Detox Shakes provide an easy way to obtain prebiotic fibers/resistant starches that play an important role in restoring health. Delaying the Detox Shakes until Day 3 gives you time to get a high-potency probiotic started that begins the process of "reseeding" the intestinal tract with healthy bacterial species, which is best started *before* your shakes begin doing their work of nourishing them. Optionally, you can also use the shakes as a means of obtaining your daily dose of iodine and vitamin D.

Coffee and teas fit into this menu plan, as does water with lemon, lime, or other non-sugary flavors. (Also see ideas for herb- and fruit-flavored drinking waters in Chapter 6.) Soft drinks, fruit juices, and carbonated beverages (except for the occasional unsweetened soda water, but not tonic water) do not fit due to excessive sugar content. And be careful with any source of alcohol: Not only do many, especially beer and whiskeys, contain wheat and grain components, but the alcohol itself has the ability to turn off your capacity to lose weight. If you'd like a drink during this process, restrict yourself to just one shot of non-grain-sourced liquor (such as grape or potato vodka or rum), one glass of dry wine, or one serving of gluten-free beer (such as Redbridge, Green's, or Bard's) per day. Your Wheat Belly 10-Day Detox is therefore a period of going very lightly with alcoholic beverages. (More detail on detox-safe alcoholic beverages can be found in Appendix B.)

Obviously, some grocery shopping will be necessary for the items required in this Menu Plan, as well as a few basic kitchen utensils. They are introduced in this chapter and listed in the Wheat Belly Detox Shopping List found in Appendix A, including a day-by-day shopping list to make the shopping process easier.

A few additional "rules" to bear in mind as you proceed through your detox:

- **Be alert when eating out.** When having a meal outside your home, you should obviously be sure to steer clear of wheat and grains. You may have to resort to the murky strategy of specifying "gluten-free" in restaurants to avoid grain contamination (for example, via utensils or work surfaces) while avoiding gluten-free breads, sauces, and desserts because of the unhealthy replacement ingredients used. If the away-from-home meal is breakfast and you miss your Detox Shake, just obtain prebiotic fibers later that day from a Detox Shake for lunch, for instance, or from another source such as a raw white potato chopped into a salad or inulin powder added to another dish.

- **Put leftovers to use.** You will inevitably have leftovers from recipes prepared from the Menu Plan that can be used for another day's meal. Leftovers work just fine and can take some of the work out of creating new dishes every day. Should you replace your morning Detox Shake with leftovers, however, or with another detox-safe dish of your choosing, just make a shake later in the day or obtain prebiotic fibers from another source.

- **Use caution when traveling.** Doing this full detox is tough if you are traveling, since the meals require home preparation. If you are confident that you can adhere to the Wheat Belly 10-Day Detox principles, however, then travel can indeed be accomplished without impairing your progress. The only allowance will be to bring some form of prebiotic fiber along (for example, inulin or FOS powder), as well as all your detox nutritional supplements. Ideally, however, you spend the 10 days of this initial and crucial process at home and try to prepare most of the recipes provided.

- **Absolutely avoid going off-program.** I've said this before, but I'll say it again: Avoid a wheat/grain "indulgence." Not only can this indulgence trigger a recurrence of unpleasant symptoms, such as bloating and diarrhea, but it will also cause you to have to start all over again, since appetite will be retriggered and all the other benefits you hoped for will be halted or reversed. From this one simple indulgence, inflammation is retriggered, water retention resumes, and joint pain and skin rashes can recur. If you desire something sweet, consult the Wheat Belly snack recipes in Chapter 6— you will enjoy your indulgence with no downside. It's not that tough, and the modest effort required to be meticulously wheat- and grain-free is truly worth it.

There are a few additional ground rules to follow in order to navigate this lifestyle effectively and to full effect. This information will provide some strategies that will help you manage this lifestyle with maximum effectiveness.

WHEAT BELLY DETOX-SAFE FLOURS AND MEALS

The meals or flours we choose for baking and breading must not contain any wheat or other grain, must be low in carbohydrates (to avoid triggering insulin that causes weight gain), and must be otherwise healthy. Choose your meals and flours by these criteria, and you can have, say, pizza, muffins, or scones that don't trigger the problems of their grain-based counterparts yet are still delicious.

Anyone with allergies to ground nuts, especially ground almonds or flour, can find several potential replacement flours in the following list. For example, sesame seeds, ground in your food processor or food chopper, yield a wonderful flour that can be used alone or combined with a small quantity of coconut flour to make any recipe that calls for almond meal or flour. (Just be careful, as some people who are allergic to nuts are also allergic to sesame and other seeds. Look for less expensive bulk sesame seeds, hulled or unhulled, not the small quantities sold in the spice aisle, and choose lighter-colored, not black or brown, varieties. Allergy to lupin flour, sourced from a legume, can also overlap with peanut allergy.) However, note that some adjustment of liquid quantity and cooking time may be required with substitutions. A wooden pick inserted into the baked dish should withdraw dry when the dish is fully cooked.

Also, garbanzo bean (chickpea) flour and coconut flour are meant to be secondary flours only (that is, used after a primary flour, such as almond or sesame seed) because the carbohydrate content of garbanzo bean flour is a bit high and coconut flour will yield too dense and dry of an end product if used alone. For example: 3 cups sesame flour + ½ cup garbanzo bean flour, or 3 cups almond flour + ¼ cup coconut flour. You will find that combining such flours or meals in this fashion improves the structure of the end product.

Choose from:

- Chia seed and flour
- Coconut flour
- Garbanzo bean (chickpea) flour
- Ground almonds and flour
- Ground golden flaxseeds
- Ground hazelnuts

- Ground peanuts and flour
- Ground pecans
- Ground psyllium seeds
- Ground pumpkin seeds
- Ground sesame seeds
- Ground sunflower seeds
- Ground walnuts
- Lupin flour

Some of these nuts/flours cannot be purchased ground and will need to be ground in a food chopper, coffee grinder, or food processor. This process usually takes about 30 to 60 seconds. Grind just until the desired texture is obtained and no more; otherwise, you'll end up with nut or seed butters.

The term *ground* refers to the end product of grinding *whole* nuts or seeds, including skins; *flour* refers to the end product from grinding *blanched* nuts with their skins removed, sometimes with the oils pressed out, yielding a finer flour texture and lighter end result after baking. Flours are the preferred form when a fine texture is desired, as in a cake. Otherwise, the less expensive meals will do just fine. Seeds will generally be ground from the whole seed, as removing the skins would be too laborious.

All flours should be stored in the refrigerator or freezer in an airtight container to slow oxidation. Alternatively, buy your nuts and seeds whole and grind only as much as you need for the recipe at hand.

Just to be absolutely clear, we avoid flours ground from:

- Wheat (white, whole wheat, whole grain, organic, sprouted), rye, barley, oat, triticale, bulgur, corn, sorghum
- Amaranth, teff, millet, chestnut, buckwheat, quinoa
- Gluten-free flours: cornflour, rice flour, potato flour, tapioca starch

WHEAT BELLY DETOX-FRIENDLY OILS

Remember: In the Wheat Belly 10-Day Detox, we *want* fats and oils in our diet. We do not cut back on fats or oils, but *increase* them. Contrary to the blundering health advice of the last half-century, fats and oils do not make you fat; they help you *lose* weight. Fats and oils do not trigger insulin, the hormone of weight gain, nor do they increase risk for cardiovascular disease. Further, they generate satiety—feeling full and satisfied. But it is best if you choose your oils wisely. Oils that were previously thought to be unhealthy, such as coconut oil and palm oil due to saturated fat content, now make a glorious return in our healthy lifestyle. We also don't trim the fat off of poultry, beef, pork, or fish, and we don't skim the gelatin and fat off our soup or stock, even when using fats like lard and tallow in our cooking (provided they are not hydrogenated by the manufacturer, if purchased).

Among the best oils to choose are:

- Avocado oil
- Butter and ghee (preferably organic)
- Coconut oil
- Extra-virgin olive oil or extra-light olive oil for baking
- Flaxseed oil
- Lard and tallow—saved from your own cooking or purchased (look for types that aren't hydrogenated)
- Macadamia oil
- Palm oil, red palm oil (preferably from sustainable sources)
- Walnut oil

There's no need to purchase each and every one of these healthy oils. You will find that just keeping a supply of coconut and extra-virgin olive oil will meet most of your cooking needs.

Consider adding healthy fats and oils at every meal opportunity: whipping melted coconut oil or butter into coffee, generously adding extra-virgin olive oil to scrambled or fried eggs, using melted coconut oil or avocado oil in your smoothie or shake. Of course, you can also feel free to savor fatty cuts of meat as well. Get more fat, and you will be able to navigate this lifestyle more smoothly.

We avoid or minimize corn oil (which also contains residues of grain proteins), vegetable oils, safflower oil, sunflower oil, grapeseed oil, and soybean oil, as they tend to weigh the diet too heavily with omega-6 oils. Though omega-6s are among the essential oils, large quantities of them are unhealthy. (The small quantity of such oils in a vitamin D capsule or other supplement is likely harmless. It's the larger intakes we are trying to avoid, such as the amount used in cooking or in processed foods.)

WHEAT BELLY DETOX-SAFE SWEETENERS

There are safe sweeteners and there are not-so-safe sweeteners that can introduce potential problems. Let's stick with the safest sweeteners of all.

The key with our choice of sweeteners is to choose the sweetener or combination of sweeteners you like most and stick with it. This way, you will be comfortable with how your sweetener behaves and tastes in various dishes, and you'll have the least surprises. Also, recall that, as you proceed through changes in taste perception during the 10-Day Detox and onward, less and less sweetener will be required. All recipes in this book that rely on safe sweeteners therefore should be adjusted to your individual taste. (This can be a special challenge, for example, if you have achieved a highly sensitive palate to sweetness, thereby requiring very little sweetener, while the family not yet following this lifestyle still desires extreme sweetness to be satisfied. You will have to choose which palate to accommodate.)

Among our top picks for safe sweeteners is stevia, a natural sweetener from the stevia plant. Unfortunately, some people experience a sharp metallic aftertaste with it. For this reason, *combining* sweeteners can be a useful strategy. Combine stevia with erythritol or monk fruit, for example, and less stevia will be

Helpful Kitchen Tools

You already have nearly all of the basic kitchen tools you will need to navigate this new lifestyle. The only new and unique utensils and equipment that would be helpful in preparing these recipes are:

- A spiral-cutting device to create spaghetti. While formerly found only in specialty cooking stores, they are now widely available and can be found in many mainstream department stores. These devices are priceless for quickly and effortlessly creating spaghetti in a variety of shapes, such as noodles or fettuccine. The Spirelli Spiral Slicer, a spiralizer, Veggetti, Benriner Spiral Cutter, and Sur La Table Vegetable and Fruit Spiral Slicer are among the most popular.

- A grinding device. While a food processor works great to grind nuts and other foods, I find that cleanup is a hassle, especially if it's used with any frequency or for small jobs, such as grinding a handful of nuts. I therefore use a food chopper to grind efficiently with quick cleanup. Even a coffee grinder can get the job done with less need for cleanup.

- A powerful blender. It helps to have a blender with a motor powerful enough not to stall when we make our Wheat Belly Detox Shakes that include ingredients like a coarsely chopped potato or green banana. A Vitamix handles these ingredients easily, though I also tried using a less powerful NutriBullet, and it handled the job without problems. If you are uncertain about the power of your blender, start by chopping your ingredients to a finer size, then see if your device handles the job. If it does, you can try increasingly larger pieces. If it doesn't, then you might consider purchasing a blender with more muscle.

- Parchment paper. Grain-free baking is made easier with a supply of parchment paper for baking pizzas and other dishes.

required and the aftertaste will be reduced or eliminated. (See Appendix B for a list of premixed sweetener combinations.)

Safe sweetener choices include:

STEVIA. Stevia is the natural sweetener from the stevia plant. Look for pure liquid stevia, pure powdered stevia, or powdered stevia with inulin; avoid stevia with maltodextrin, since maltodextrin is a form of sugar. My favorite is pure powdered stevia; though pricey, it is so concentrated that a tiny amount goes a long way and a container will last a while.

MONK FRUIT. Also known as lo han guo, monk fruit is a rising star in the world of benign sweeteners. A growing number of people like this sweetener due to its clean, sweet taste without the aftertaste some people perceive with stevia. It may be tricky to find but is becoming increasingly available.

ERYTHRITOL. Erythritol is a natural sweetener found in fruit that has approximately 70 percent of the sweetness of sugar. Taking into account your increasing sensitivity to sweetness, you can use erythritol, spoonful for spoonful, just as you would sugar. It is especially useful combined with stevia.

XYLITOL. Xylitol is the most sugarlike of our choice of sweeteners and can be useful for glazing and streusel effects in baking. We use xylitol only in limited quantities, however, because it has a modest capacity to raise blood sugar. And dog owners should know that xylitol can be toxic to dogs.

INULIN. Inulin is a fiber with a light sweetness that is best used in combination with other sweeteners. It also acts as a prebiotic fiber or resistant starch that can, unlike other forms of such fibers, be resistant to heating and not degrade to sugars.

THE WHEAT BELLY 10-DAY DETOX MENU PLAN

While there's nothing fancy or complicated in this Menu Plan— no *rillette de canard* nor other tongue-twisting French gourmet dishes here—I believe that you will nonetheless enjoy putting these recipes together while gaining the incredible benefits of eating without the health impairment from grains.

We need to bear in mind that energy and motivation may hit a low point as you proceed through your wheat and grain withdrawal process. You may find that even the easiest, most common tasks, such as getting the kids off to school or keeping up with your social schedule, seem impossibly demanding, let alone having to put together an entirely new menu. The recipes provided are therefore simple, tasty, and consistent with Wheat Belly principles, placing as little strain as possible on top of your early detoxification experience while providing maximum benefit.

You will be pleasantly surprised with the variety of flavors you'll experience when eating without grains, especially as you reacquire the heightened sense of taste that typically develops over the first few days to weeks of grain detoxification. I recognize that you may be the primary meal preparer in the family, so I've also included recipes that are spouse-friendly and kid-friendly. To expand your arsenal of recipes to satisfy the family, you can also supplement family meals with dishes using the recipes in Chapters 6 and 7. Feel free to use these additional recipes anytime during your detox experience, as well as afterward, if you are up to the task.

As you proceed through your 10-Day Menu Plan, you will see that we make no effort to reduce fat, pour off excess oils, limit calories or portions, or other unnecessary, even counterproductive, maneuvers. These are not oversights—they're intentional. While most people experience a dramatic reduction in appetite within the 10 days of their detox, we do not purposefully reduce or count calories—it will happen naturally and effortlessly, especially if you augment the amount of healthy fats and oils in your diet. So even if a dish on this menu is packed with fat and calories (as many are), *nobody* should be sweating these issues—eat it, enjoy it.

Most of the dishes are prepared from "scratch," meaning some extra effort is involved compared to just microwaving a frozen dinner. This is also intentional, as it is difficult to obtain truly healthy foods that are preprepared. You can also eat with greater confidence when you control the ingredients. A few time-saving foods are used, such as prepared mayonnaise and tomato sauce, but just be sure to examine the label for problem ingredients, though it is always an option to make your own. (A recipe for Homemade Marinara Sauce is included on page 121. Recipes for healthy homemade mayonnaise and other condiments and sauces can be found in the *Wheat Belly 30-Minute Cookbook*.)

I recognize that there is effort involved in preparing these recipes that can pose special challenges while you are wallowing in the throes of your wheat and grain withdrawal and struggling with fatigue. Should you not be up to the task for a meal or for a day, you can substitute easier dishes, perhaps one you've prepared

---

ELIZABETH, 48, sales consultant, New York

During her detox, Elizabeth experienced headaches, reduced energy, and very little stamina until Day 5. "My joint pain was on and off, but a bit better. My stomach wasn't as bloated or fat.

"I noticed a difference in my pain level once I started removing the wheat and sugar. During the detox, I took a very long walk (around 2 hours, more than 5 miles). I was tired, but I made it through the walk. This is something that I would definitely struggle with previously. I had this weird rash or eczema type of thing around my neck. My skin was red, dry, and irritated in a ring just where my hairline hit my neck. That has completely disappeared. My energy level is really good; I rarely get tired during the day at all, and I sleep really well at night."

By the end of her 10-day experience, Elizabeth had lost the most of all our detox participants: 13.2 pounds, or 6 percent of her starting body weight.

in the past without a recipe, such as an omelet for breakfast or just a simple steak and salad for dinner, or use the leftovers from prior Detox Menu Plan recipes. Just be sure to adhere to the rule of no wheat or grains, limiting carbohydrate exposure to no more than 15 grams net carbs per meal, and carefully choose products such as salad dressing that are free of problem grain and sugar ingredients (use olive oil and vinegar, for instance, or salsa, pico de gallo, infused olive oils, or other safe products). This way, you can have your meal and not impair your progress. Once again, if you choose to skip your Detox Shake for breakfast, just include it later in the day or use an alternative source of prebiotic fibers.

For most of the lunches and dinners, I've provided the main dish or stand-alone dish by itself; feel free to add a steamed vegetable or green salad as often as you like to increase your veggie intake.

DAY 1

BREAKFAST
Apricot Ginger "Granola" (page 108)

LUNCH
Cream of Broccoli Soup (page 109)

DINNER
Italian Sausage and Pepper Pizza (pages 110–111)

DAY 2

BREAKFAST
Berry Coconut Quick Muffin (page 112)

LUNCH
Egg salad or ham/turkey/beef with mayonnaise or mustard on Wheat Belly Herbed Focaccia Bread (page 113)

DINNER
Aubergine Lasagna (pages 114–115)

Green salad with olive oil and balsamic vinegar

DAY 3

BREAKFAST
Wheat Belly Detox Shake (flavor of your choice) (pages 104–107). Use only half of the green banana or raw potato called for in the recipe.

LUNCH
Mediterranean "Pasta" Salad (page 116)

DINNER
Bacon-Topped Meat Loaf with Mushrooms and Gravy (page 117)

Mashed "Potatoes" (page 118) and green beans

DAY 4

BREAKFAST
Wheat Belly Detox Shake (flavor of your choice) (pages
104–107). Use only half of the green banana or raw potato
called for in the recipe.

LUNCH
Spicy Italian Frittata (page 119)

DINNER
Spaghetti with Meatballs (page 120)

Baked olive oil–coated asparagus

DAY 5

BREAKFAST
Wheat Belly Detox Shake (flavor of your choice) (pages
104–107). Use only half of the green banana or raw potato
called for in the recipe.

LUNCH
Curried Chicken Soup (page 122)

DINNER
Fettuccine Alfredo (page 123) with steamed broccoli

Chocolate Avocado Pudding (page 124)

DAY 6

BREAKFAST
Wheat Belly Detox Shake (flavor of your choice) (pages 104–107). Use only half of the green banana or raw potato called for in the recipe.

LUNCH
Aubergine Mini Pizzas (page 125)

DINNER
Pork Thai Stir-Fry (page 126)

DAY 7

BREAKFAST
Wheat Belly Detox Shake (flavor of your choice) (pages 104–107). Use only half of the green banana or raw potato called for in the recipe.

LUNCH
Chorizo, Pepper, and Avocado Fry-Up (page 127)

DINNER
Bacon-Wrapped Chicken Breasts Stuffed with Spinach, Mushrooms, and Roasted Red Peppers (page 128)

Green salad or vegetable side dish of your choice, such as steamed broccoli or green beans

DAY 8

BREAKFAST
Wheat Belly Detox Shake (flavor of your choice) (pages 104–107). Use only half of the green banana or raw potato called for in the recipe.

LUNCH
Spicy Minestrone (page 129)

DINNER
Prawn Fried "Rice" (page 130)

DAY 9

BREAKFAST
Wheat Belly Detox Shake (flavor of your choice) (pages 104–107). Begin to use an entire green banana or raw potato.

LUNCH
Jumbo Gingerbread Nut Muffin (page 131)

DINNER
Bratwurst with Peppers and Sauerkraut (page 132)

"Potato" Salad (page 133)

DAY 10

BREAKFAST
Wheat Belly Detox Shake (flavor of your choice) (pages 104–107). Use an entire green banana or raw potato.

LUNCH
BLT Wrap (pages 134–135)

DINNER
Roasted Brussels Sprouts and Ham Fry-Up (page 136)

RECIPES

WHEAT BELLY DETOX SHAKES

These are no ordinary shakes. Wheat Belly Detox Shakes give you that extra boost to accelerate success in losing weight and undoing the harmful effects previously incurred by eating wheat and grains. They are also easy to prepare, delicious, and surprisingly filling.

Detox Shakes come in a variety of flavors and serve as a source of prebiotic fibers to nourish bowel flora. One Detox Shake per day provides your entire daily intake required to cultivate and nourish healthy bowel flora. Remember: A transition back to a healthier profile of bowel flora is part of the formula for success in this lifestyle because it furthers the health and metabolic benefits of wheat and grain elimination. When combined with the probiotic strategy discussed earlier, it cultivates the bowel flora diversity that is a marker for great health, and helps minimize or avoid disruptions in bowel habits, such as constipation and bloating, that can develop during the first few weeks of dietary changes. Note that you ideally *vary* the source of prebiotic fibers/resistant starches by using, for example, a green banana in your shake on Monday, a raw potato on Tuesday, etc., as this encourages species diversity in bowel flora, a feature that characterizes high levels of overall health. Recall that the healthiest, slenderest, most metabolically healthy people have the greatest species diversity, i.e., the widest number of healthy species in their intestines. Varying your source of prebiotic fibers from day to day encourages species diversity.

The healthy fats of the coconut oil in each shake induce satiety for many hours afterward. These shakes are filling so that they easily can be consumed as stand-alone meals or meal replacements. They can also be used alongside a meal, but they truly are very filling and will reduce your need for other foods. Should you desire an even *more* filling meal replacement, add the pulp of one avocado, though you'll have to add 110 ml (4 fl oz) or more water or other safe liquid (e.g., more unsweetened coconut milk) to keep it drinkable rather than spoonable. But be warned: You will have an exceptionally filling meal that, if consumed for breakfast, may take you all the way to dinner and beyond.

The shakes are designed to make a substantial contribution to your daily requirement of magnesium from seeds. If pumpkin seeds are used, the shake adds 190 milligrams of (elemental) magnesium to your diet, while sunflower seeds add 117 milligrams. (It still helps to take a magnesium supplement as discussed in the previous chapter.) An occasional person, in the midst of detoxifying and staging a gastrointestinal recovery from grains, encounters difficulty with the quantity of seeds in the Detox Shakes; if you experience discomfort, leave out the seeds during this early experience. The inclusion of coconut milk, green banana or raw potato, and the optional avocado also yields oodles of potassium that helps maintain bone health and makes a major contribution to controlling blood pressure.

Each shake variation can also be used to obtain unique health benefits: metabolic improvements, such as reduced blood pressure, from a big wallop of cocoa polyphenols in the Mocha Coconut Detox Shake; metabolic benefits and modestly enhanced weight loss from the Green Tea Ginger Detox Shake; anti-inflammatory benefits from the Tropical Storm Detox Shake; and blood sugar benefits from plentiful Ceylon cinnamon in the Cinnamon Apple Pie Detox Shake. Choose the shake flavor and/or benefit you like best, or vary from day to day.

I advise you to use a blender or food processor/chopper with a strong motor, strong enough to handle the tough green unripe banana or raw potato. Note that the banana must be *green and unripe*, providing fibers that are indigestible to humans but digestible by bowel flora. One medium green, unripe banana yields up to 27 grams of indigestible fiber, while one medium (9 cm/3½ inches in length) raw potato yields 20 grams. Recall that we aim for a total prebiotic fiber intake of 20 grams per day, a target not achieved in our Detox Shakes until Day 9 and 10. We therefore start with half a banana or half a potato, or no more than 10 to 13 grams of indigestible fiber per day, on Day 3, then increase to a whole banana or potato on Day 9. If you jump to the whole banana or potato too soon, you may experience excessive bloating and abdominal discomfort. It is also important that you start taking your high-potency probiotic supplement beginning on Day 1 to "seed" your intestines with healthy species.

Note that if you experience abdominal discomfort with these shakes, you may need to stop and consult your doctor since this suggests that bowel flora may be severely disrupted from your previous diet and will not normalize with these simple, natural efforts. Thankfully, this is uncommon, but it's critical to correct; correction may require an initial period of prescription antibiotics and/or other corrective strategies to eliminate the undesirable bacterial species that have dominated your bowel flora and begin with a clean "slate." Functional medicine practitioners and naturopaths are most likely to be expert in this area.

Optionally, these shakes can be used as a means of supplementing liquid iodine and vitamin D drops. The optional vitamin D dose suggested can be adjusted to suit individual needs; because 5,000 international units (IU) is a common need for adult men and women, I listed this as the quantity in the recipes below, but this amount can be adjusted to your individual need. Likewise, 500 micrograms of iodine is specified, as I believe this is close to an ideal dose, but you may need to adjust your iodine intake to your individual needs.

You can further modify your shakes by adding, for instance, a teaspoon or two of inulin powder to supplement the prebiotic fiber content; spinach, chard, kale, or spirulina for a dose of green veggies; and other vitamins, minerals, or nutrients.

MOCHA COCONUT DETOX SHAKE

Cocoa in the form of cocoa powder is the most concentrated source of cocoa poly-phenols that yield all the health benefits of cocoa and chocolate, including modest reductions in insulin and blood pressure and reduced cardiovascular risk. You can enjoy cocoa without guilt, as there is no added sugar to botch things up. An easy variation is to omit the coffee granules and replace them with 2 tablespoons of unsweetened, natural peanut butter to create a peanut butter cup flavor.

Makes 1

1 medium green banana or medium peeled raw white potato

60 ml (2 fl oz) coconut oil, melted

240 ml (8 fl oz) unsweetened coconut, almond, or hemp milk

120 ml (4 fl oz) water

30 g (1 oz) raw pumpkin or sunflower seeds

Sweetener equivalent to 1 tablespoon sugar (e.g., ¼ teaspoon pure powdered stevia)

2½ tablespoons unsweetened cocoa powder

1 teaspoon instant coffee granules

½ teaspoon vanilla extract

Potassium iodide drops or kelp powder to provide 500 mcg iodine; liquid vitamin D drops to provide 5,000 IU (optional)

If using a green banana, peel and coarsely chop it. It's easier to use a knife and cut the peel lengthwise first, then shell out the pulp. If using a potato, coarsely chop it. In a blender, combine the banana or potato, coconut oil, milk, water, seeds, sweetener, cocoa, coffee granules, vanilla, and iodine source and vitamin D (if using). Blend until well mixed and the banana or potato have been liquefied. Serve immediately.

If your shake is too thick, add 60 ml (2 fl oz) of water and blend briefly to mix.

Note: *Don't be fooled by the apparent high-carbohydrate count in these Detox Shakes. The carb grams quoted include the prebiotic fibers from the green banana or raw potato.*

Per serving: 911 calories, 18 g protein, 36 g carbohydrates, 82 g total fat, 55 g saturated fat, 9 g fiber, 32 mg sodium

GREEN TEA GINGER DETOX SHAKE

The polyphenols in green tea, as with cocoa, provide modest health benefits including reduced blood pressure, reduced insulin and blood sugar, facilitation of weight loss, and reduced fatty liver that typically accompanies a wheat belly. The powdered green tea used in this shake provides a wallop of green tea polyphenols because, unlike brewed tea in which the nutrients are extracted with hot water, you are actually consuming the powdered, ground tea leaves. You can find powdered matcha green tea in Asian food stores.

Makes 1

1 medium green banana or medium peeled raw white potato

60 ml (2 fl oz) coconut oil, melted

240 ml (8 fl oz) unsweetened coconut, almond, or hemp milk

120 ml (4 fl oz) water

30 g (1 oz) raw pumpkin or sunflower seeds

Sweetener equivalent to 1 tablespoon sugar (e.g., ¼ teaspoon pure powdered stevia)

1 teaspoon powdered matcha green tea

½ teaspoon ground ginger

Potassium iodide drops or kelp powder to provide 500 mcg iodine; liquid vitamin D drops to provide 5,000 IU (optional)

If using a green banana, peel and coarsely chop it. It's easier to use a knife and cut the peel lengthwise first, then shell out the pulp. If using a potato, coarsely chop it. In a blender, combine the banana or potato, coconut oil, milk, water, seeds, sweetener, green tea, ginger, and iodine source and vitamin D (if using). Blend until well mixed and the banana or potato have been liquefied. Serve immediately.

If your shake is too thick, add 60 ml (2 fl oz) of water and blend briefly to mix.

Note: *Don't be fooled by the apparent high-carbohydrate count in these Detox Shakes. The carb grams quoted include the prebiotic fibers from the green banana or raw potato.*

Per serving: 892 calories, 16 g protein, 30 g carbohydrates, 81 g total fat, 55 g saturated fat, 4 g fiber, 39 mg sodium

Variation:
Replace the ground ginger with a mint leaf or 30 g (1 oz) of raspberries.

TROPICAL STORM DETOX SHAKE

This Tropical Storm Shake, as its name suggests, provides the refreshing tropical flavors of coconut and pineapple while providing a modest quantity of turmeric, a source of curcumin, which exerts anti-inflammatory and cancer-preventing effects. Ginger can also add to the anti-inflammatory benefits. The quantity of turmeric specified provides approximately 90 milligrams of active curcumin. (Additional anti-inflammatory benefits can be obtained by taking curcumin supplements, typically at a dose of 500 milligrams twice per day, a dosage that has been shown to yield modest benefits in rheumatoid arthritis, ulcerative colitis, and Crohn's disease, as well as prevention of cancer and dementia.)

Makes 1

1 medium green banana or medium peeled raw white potato

60 ml (2 fl oz) coconut oil, melted

240 ml (8 fl oz) unsweetened coconut, almond, or hemp milk

120 ml (4 fl oz) water

30 g (1 oz) raw pumpkin or sunflower seeds

Sweetener equivalent to 1 tablespoon sugar (e.g., ¼ teaspoon pure powdered stevia)

15 g (½ oz) unsweetened shredded coconut

40 g (1½ oz) fresh chopped pineapple

1½ teaspoons ground turmeric

½ teaspoon ground ginger

Potassium iodide drops or kelp powder to provide 500 mcg iodine; liquid vitamin D drops to provide 5,000 IU (optional)

If using a green banana, peel and coarsely chop it. It's easier to use a knife and cut the peel lengthwise first, then shell out the pulp. If using a potato, coarsely chop it. In a blender, combine the banana or potato, coconut oil, milk, water, seeds, sweetener, coconut, pineapple, turmeric, ginger, and iodine source and vitamin D (if using). Blend until well mixed and the banana or potato have been liquefied. Serve immediately.

If your shake is too thick, add 60 ml (2 fl oz) of water and blend briefly to mix.

Note: *Don't be fooled by the apparent high-carbohydrate count in these Detox Shakes. The carb grams quoted include the prebiotic fibers from the green banana or raw potato.*

Per serving: 1,069 calories, 17 g protein, 40 g carbohydrates, 96 g total fat, 68 g saturated fat, 8 g fiber, 40 mg sodium

CINNAMON APPLE PIE DETOX SHAKE

If you desire the potential health benefits of cinnamon, such as modest reductions in blood sugar, choose the Ceylon variety that has been associated with such benefits. (Cassia, Viet Nam, Saigon, and Chinese cinnamons are flavorful and fragrant, but they lack the health benefits.) Specialty spice stores, gourmet shops, or health food stores are your best bets as sources.

Makes 1

1 medium green banana or medium peeled raw white potato

65g (2½ oz) unsweetened apple purée

60 ml (2 fl oz) coconut oil, melted

240 ml (8 fl oz) unsweetened coconut, almond, or hemp milk

120 ml (4 fl oz) water

30 g (1 oz) raw pumpkin or sunflower seeds

Sweetener equivalent to 1 tablespoon sugar (e.g., ¼ teaspoon pure powdered stevia)

1½ teaspoons ground Ceylon cinnamon

½ teaspoon vanilla extract

Potassium iodide drops or kelp powder to provide 500 mcg iodine; liquid vitamin D drops to provide 5,000 IU (optional)

If using a green banana, peel and coarsely chop it. It's easier to use a knife and cut the peel lengthwise first, then shell out the pulp. If using a potato, coarsely chop it. In a blender, combine the banana or potato, apple purée, coconut oil, milk, water, seeds, sweetener, cinnamon, vanilla, and iodine source and vitamin D (if using). Blend until well mixed and the banana or potato have been liquefied. Serve immediately.

If your shake is too thick, add 60 ml (2 fl oz) of water and blend briefly to mix.

Note: *Don't be fooled by the apparent high-carbohydrate count in these Detox Shakes. The carb grams quoted include the prebiotic fibers from the green banana or raw potato.*

Per serving: 918 calories, 16 g protein, 38 g carbohydrates, 81 g total fat, 55 g saturated fat, 7 g fiber, 33 mg sodium

DAY 1

APRICOT GINGER "GRANOLA"

Here's your answer to breakfast cereal—but this "granola" has *none* of the problems of the products that line an entire aisle at your supermarket. Serve this granola mix with unsweetened coconut milk or almond milk, cold or hot.

This recipe makes use of a modest quantity of fruit sugar from apricots. If it's not sweet enough for, say, your 7-year-old, a few raisins sprinkled on top or a bit of stevia or your choice of sweetener can be added. The use of dried apricots allows you to minimize the use of the sweetener, while adding only around 20 grams of net carbohydrates to the entire batch.

Use leftovers as a snack. This granola can be stored in an airtight container at room temperature and will keep for about a week.

Makes 10 servings

5 dried apricots

60 ml (2 fl oz) coconut oil, melted

2 teaspoons vanilla extract

½ teaspoon almond extract

250 g (9 oz) raw sunflower seeds

250 g (9 oz) raw pumpkin seeds

125 g (4½ oz) chopped raw pecans

90g (3 oz) flaked raw almonds

175 g (6 oz) unsweetened coconut flakes or shredded unsweetened coconut

1 teaspoon ground ginger

1 teaspoon ground allspice

Sweetener equivalent to 55 g (2 oz) cup sugar (optional)

Preheat the oven to 140°C/275°F/Gas mark 1.

In a food processor or food chopper, pulse the apricots until they're reduced to very small fragments. In a small bowl, combine the apricots and coconut oil and mix thoroughly. Add the vanilla and almond extract and stir. Set aside.

In a large bowl, combine the sunflower seeds, pumpkin seeds, pecans, almonds, coconut, ginger, allspice, and sweetener (if using). Stir in the reserved apricot mixture until well mixed.

Spread the mixture in a large baking pan and bake for about 15 minutes, stirring halfway through, or until lightly browned. Remove and cool.

Per serving: 702 calories, 18 g protein, 21 g carbohydrates, 61 g total fat, 25 g saturated fat, 9 g fiber, 14 mg sodium

CREAM OF BROCCOLI SOUP

With the use of a blender, this wonderfully filling and simple variation on traditional cream of broccoli soup can be whipped up in just a few minutes. We put coconut milk to use to take advantage of its satiating and other health effects; it also makes this soup so tasty that you'll want to lick the spoon.

Makes 6 servings

60 g (2½ oz) butter, coconut oil, or extra-virgin olive oil

1 medium onion, chopped

2 cloves garlic, minced

1 litre chicken stock

450 g (1 lb) fresh or frozen broccoli florets

1 can (440 ml/14 fl oz) coconut milk

1 teaspoon sea salt

¼ teaspoon ground black pepper

In a large pot over medium-high heat, heat the butter or oil. Cook the onion and garlic until the onion is translucent. Increase the heat to high and add the stock. Bring the mixture to a boil, then reduce the heat to medium. Add the broccoli, coconut milk, salt, and pepper and cook, stirring occasionally, for 5 minutes, or until the broccoli is softened.

Pour the mixture into a blender and blend until smooth. Alternatively, a handheld immersion blender can be used.

Per serving: 286 calories, 8 g protein, 14 g carbohydrates, 24 g total fat, 18 g saturated fat, 3 g fiber, 588 mg sodium

ITALIAN SAUSAGE AND PEPPER PIZZA

I purposely put this tasty pizza dish on your first day's menu. Even though it involves some preparation, you will be rewarded with a delicious pizza that will convince you and your family members that living the Wheat Belly way is rich and tasty!

If there are leftovers, you can save them for tomorrow's breakfast.

Makes 8 servings

250 g (9 oz) ground almonds/ flour

300 g (11 oz) shredded mozzarella cheese, divided

30 g (1 oz) ground golden flaxseeds

1 teaspoon onion powder

½ teaspoon sea salt

2 large eggs

120 ml (4 fl oz) extra-virgin olive oil, divided

120 ml (4 fl oz) water

225 g (8 oz) Italian sausage, loose or removed from casing

1 onion, chopped

2 cloves garlic, minced

1 small red pepper, seeded and sliced

1 small green or yellow pepper, seeded and sliced

250 g (9 oz) pizza sauce

¼ teaspoon crushed red chillies

¼ teaspoon salt

⅛ teaspoon ground black pepper

Preheat the oven to 180°C/350°F/Gas mark 4.

In a large bowl, combine the ground almonds/flour, half the cheese, the flaxseeds, onion powder, and sea salt and mix well.

In a small bowl, whisk the eggs. Add half the olive oil and the water. Pour the egg mixture into the ground almonds/flour mixture and combine thoroughly.

Spread parchment paper over a pizza pan or baking sheet. Place the dough on the parchment paper. Coat your hands in olive oil and form the dough by hand into a 30 cm (12 in) diameter round or other desired shape. Alternatively, place a second sheet of parchment paper on top of the dough and flatten with a rolling pin into the desired shape and size; feel around the edges to gauge thickness. Remove the top layer of parchment paper carefully. Use a spatula or spoon to form the crust edge.

Bake for 20 minutes.

Meanwhile, in a large frying pan over medium-high heat, heat 1 tablespoon olive oil. Cook the sausage until no longer pink. Add the onion, garlic, and peppers and cook, stirring occasionally, until the onion is translucent and the peppers have softened. Remove from the heat.

Remove the pizza crust from the oven and spread with the pizza sauce. Top with the sausage mixture, remaining cheese, and remaining 3 tablespoons olive oil. Add the crushed chillies, salt, and black pepper. Bake for 10 minutes, or until the cheese has melted.

Per serving: 514 calories, 22 g protein, 15 g carbohydrates, 43 g total fat, 8 g saturated fat, 6 g fiber, 599 mg sodium

DAY 2

BERRY COCONUT QUICK MUFFIN

Quick muffins are single-serve muffins prepared in a mug or ramekin, minimizing preparation and cleanup time and perfect for a quick, on-the-run, healthy breakfast in the morning. While the directions call for cooking in a microwave, quick muffins can also be made in the oven using an ovenproof ramekin; bake the muffin at 190°C/375°F/Gas mark 5 for 15 minutes. As always, taste your batter before microwaving or baking to gauge sweetness and adjust as desired.

Makes 1

55 g (2 oz) ground almonds/flour

15 g (½ oz) shredded unsweetened coconut

1 teaspoon ground cinnamon

Sweetener equivalent to 1 tablespoon sugar

2 eggs

2 tablespoons coconut oil, melted

55 g (2 oz) fresh or frozen mixed berries

In a large mug or ramekin, combine the ground almonds/flour, coconut, cinnamon, and sweetener. Add the eggs and coconut oil and mix well. Gently stir in the berries.

Microwave on high power for 2½ minutes, or until cooked through. (If using fresh berries, a shorter time is required, typically 30 seconds less.)

Per serving: 884 calories, 26 g protein, 25 g carbohydrates, 80 g total fat, 41 g saturated fat, 11 g fiber, 169 mg sodium

WHEAT BELLY HERBED FOCACCIA BREAD

Here is a quick, virtually foolproof flatbread that gets around the somewhat tricky effort to create "rise" in grain-free baking. Although this bread recipe is included to allow you to make the occasional sandwich, you may find this bread tasty enough to eat as is, or just dipped in extra-virgin olive oil sprinkled with some kosher or sea salt.

Makes 6 servings

150 g (5 oz) shredded mozzarella or other cheese

300 g (11 oz) ground almonds/flour

1½ teaspoons sea salt or kosher salt, divided

1 teaspoon onion powder

½ teaspoon garlic powder

1½ teaspoons dried rosemary

1½ teaspoons dried oregano

80 g (3 oz) black or kalamata olives, finely chopped or sliced

40 g (1½ oz) sun-dried tomatoes, finely sliced

2 large eggs

120 ml (4 fl oz) extra-virgin olive oil, divided

Preheat the oven to 190°C/375°F/Gas mark 5.

In a medium bowl, combine the cheese, ground almonds/flour, ½ teaspoon of the salt, the onion powder, garlic powder, rosemary, oregano, olives, and tomatoes and mix together. Set aside.

In a small bowl, whisk the eggs. Add all but 1 tablespoon of the olive oil and stir to combine. Pour the egg mixture into the reserved ground almonds/flour mixture and mix thoroughly.

Grease a 43 × 28 cm (17 × 11 in) shallow baking pan. Place the dough on the pan and shape into a large rectangle by hand or by covering the dough with parchment paper and using a rolling pin to roll to a 1 cm (½ in) thickness. The dough may not fill the entire pan.

Bake for 12 minutes. Remove from the oven and use the blunt handle of a wooden spoon or other small rounded utensil to make small depressions in the surface every inch or so. Brush the surface with the remaining 1 tablespoon olive oil and sprinkle with the remaining 1 teaspoon salt. Bake for 8 to 10 minutes, or until lightly browned.

Using a pizza cutter, slice the bread into 6 pieces.

Per serving: 634 calories, 21 g protein, 13 g carbohydrates, 56 g total fat, 8 g saturated fat, 7 g fiber, 624 mg sodium

AUBERGINE LASAGNA

Rich and satisfying, this Aubergine Lasagna will make you forget you ever made the recipe before using grains.

As a time-saver, this recipe uses jarred marinara sauce, so choose the brand with the least sugar added, and certainly no high-fructose corn syrup. Nowadays, you can find many brands with no more than 10 to 12 grams of net carbs per 225 g (8 oz) on most store shelves. If you'd prefer to make your own sauce, see the Homemade Tomato Sauce recipe on page 121.

Makes 8 servings

2 medium aubergines

2 tablespoons sea salt

240 ml (8fl oz) extra-virgin olive oil, divided

2 jars (375 g /13 oz) marinara sauce

2 tablespoons chopped fresh basil or 2 teaspoons dried

7g (¼ oz) chopped fresh oregano or 1 tablespoon dried

450g (1 lb) ricotta cheese

50 g (2 oz) grated Parmesan cheese

1 large egg

450 g (1 lb) mozzarella cheese, sliced or shredded

With a sharp knife, remove the ends of the aubergines, then slice lengthwise into 5 mm (¼ in) slices. (These thinner slices will brown more readily and yield more tender "noodles.") Cut the larger slices from the center in half to make narrower noodles. In a colander over the sink, toss the aubergine slices with the salt; let sit for at least 30 minutes to allow the water to drain.

Rinse the aubergine slices briefly to remove excess salt. Drain. In a large frying pan over medium-high heat, heat 2 tablespoons of the olive oil. Add aubergine slices in a single layer and cook for 2 to 3 minutes per side, or until lightly browned. (Several batches will be required; add additional oil as needed.) Set aside.

In a medium saucepan over medium heat, combine the marinara sauce, basil, and oregano. Simmer, stirring occasionally, for 5 minutes, or until heated through. Do not boil.

Preheat the oven to 190°C/375°F/Gas mark 5.

In a medium bowl, combine the ricotta, Parmesan, and egg and mix thoroughly.

Arrange 1 layer of aubergine in a 32 × 23 cm (13 × 9 in) baking dish. Top with the cheese mixture. Spread about half of the marinara sauce over the cheese layer. Top with the remaining aubergine, followed by the remaining marinara sauce. Sprinkle the top with the mozzarella.

Bake for 45 minutes, or until heated through and the cheese is golden.

Per serving: 632 calories, 24 g protein, 19 g carbohydrates, 51 g total fat, 17 g saturated fat, 6 g fiber, 1,044 mg sodium

DAY 3

MEDITERRANEAN "PASTA" SALAD

This recipe introduces spiral-cut courgettes, what some call courgetti because of their resemblance to spaghetti. You will need one of the inexpensive spiral-cutting devices, such as a Spirelli, Spiralizer, or one of the many others now on the market. While you could make do with a knife or mandoline, the spiral cutters are so much easier and quicker to use and generate thinner, more spaghetti-like slices. If you plan on having these "spaghetti" dishes with any regularity, it is well worth the modest investment.

Shorter spaghetti works best in this dish; spiral-cut the courgettes with short strokes to create lengths that are no more than 4–5 cm (1½ to 2 in). The flavors in this "pasta" salad are highlighted by the herbs, so choose fresh herbs whenever possible.

Makes 8 servings

450 g (1 lb) courgettes, spiral-cut with short strokes

225 g (8 oz) cherry tomatoes, halved

1 medium cucumber, quartered and sliced

5–6 spring onions, finely sliced

80 g (3 oz) black or kalamata olives, pitted, halved or sliced

225 g (8 oz) pepperoni, quartered and sliced

2 tablespoons chopped fresh basil or 2 teaspoons dried

1 tablespoon chopped fresh oregano or 1 teaspoon dried

60 ml (2 fl oz) white vinegar

60 ml (2 fl oz) extra-virgin olive oil

25 g (1 oz) grated Parmesan or Romano cheese (optional)

In a large bowl, combine the courgetti, tomatoes, cucumber, spring onions, olives, pepperoni, basil, oregano, vinegar, and olive oil and toss until well mixed. Top with cheese, if using.

Per serving: 240 calories, 8 g protein, 5 g carbohydrates, 21 g total fat, 5 g saturated fat, 2 g fiber, 569 mg sodium

BACON-TOPPED MEAT LOAF WITH MUSHROOMS AND GRAVY

Here's a classic recipe tweaked to fit into the Wheat Belly lifestyle; I've replaced the bread crumbs found in traditional meat loaf with ground golden flaxseeds. I also introduce you to the useful practice of thickening gravy with coconut flour, rather than wheat flour or cornflour.

Save any leftovers for sandwiches served on Wheat Belly Herbed Focaccia Bread (see page 113).

Makes 8 servings

450 g (1 lb) minced beef

450 g (1 lb) minced pork

2 eggs

65 g (2½ oz) ground golden flaxseeds

310 g (11 oz) shredded carrots

1 medium onion, chopped

1 green pepper, seeded and chopped

1 teaspoon sea salt

½ teaspoon ground black pepper

4 rashers bacon (preferably uncured)

2 tablespoons extra-virgin olive oil, coconut oil, or butter

110 g (4 oz) button mushrooms, sliced

240 ml (8 fl oz) beef stock

55 g (2 oz) coconut flour

Preheat the oven to 180°C/350°F/Gas mark 4.

In a large bowl, combine the beef, pork, eggs, flaxseeds, carrots, onion, pepper, salt, and black pepper and mix thoroughly. Spread evenly into a 32 × 23 cm (13 × 9 in) baking dish or shape into a loaf about 6 cm (2½ in) high. Lay the bacon rashers over the top. Cover with foil and bake for 1 hour.

Meanwhile, in a medium frying pan over medium-high heat, heat the oil or butter. Cook the mushrooms, stirring frequently, until lightly browned and softened. Remove from the heat and set aside.

After the meat loaf has cooked for 1 hour, remove the foil and carefully pour the drippings into the frying pan with the mushrooms. Return the meat loaf to the oven, uncovered, and cook for 30 minutes, or until a thermometer inserted in the center registers 71°C (160°F) and the meat is no longer pink.

Place the mushroom mixture over low heat and stir in the stock. Add the coconut flour, 1 tablespoon per minute, stirring frequently, until the desired thickness is obtained. Add additional salt and pepper to taste. Slice the meat loaf and serve topped with the gravy.

Per serving: 385 calories, 30 g protein, 12 g carbohydrates, 25 g total fat, 8 g saturated fat, 6 g fiber, 531 mg sodium

MASHED "POTATOES"

Although not a grain, potatoes yield too many carbohydrates when cooked. This is a problem in your 10-Day Detox because excessive carbohydrates turn off your capacity to lose weight by triggering blood sugar and insulin to high levels. Rather than simply subtracting another common staple from your dinner table, here is a way to not just replace mashed potatoes, but to create something that tastes *even better*, but with none of the problems. Replace butter with extra-virgin olive oil for a dairy-free version.

Makes 4 servings

1 large head cauliflower, cut into florets

60 ml (2 fl oz) canned coconut milk

2 tablespoons butter

¼ teaspoon sea salt

Ground black pepper to taste

Place a steamer basket in a large pot with 5 cm (2 in) of water. Bring to a boil, then reduce the heat to medium. Place the cauliflower in the basket, cover, and steam for 15 to 20 minutes, or until soft.

Remove from the heat and drain. In a blender, food processor, or food chopper, combine the cauliflower, coconut milk, butter, salt, and pepper. Blend or process until smooth.

Per serving: 131 calories, 4 g protein, 11 g carbohydrates, 9 g total fat, 6 g saturated fat, 4 g fiber, 214 mg sodium

DAY 4

SPICY ITALIAN FRITTATA

Here's a heavy-duty frittata that can fit into any meal. This Spicy Italian Frittata is used in this menu plan as a lunch dish, but it can fit just about anywhere.

Makes 6 servings

1 medium onion, chopped

2 cloves garlic, minced

225 g (8 oz) Italian sausage, loose or sliced

60 g (2½ oz) spinach leaves or kale

1 red pepper, seeded and chopped

1 teaspoon sea salt

⅛ teaspoon ground black pepper

10 eggs

2 teaspoons hot-pepper sauce

Preheat the oven to 190°C/375°F/Gas mark 5.

In a large ovenproof frying pan over medium-high heat, cook the onion, garlic, and sausage, stirring frequently, until the onion is translucent and the sausage is no longer pink. Stir in the spinach or kale, pepper, salt, and black pepper and cook, covered, stirring occasionally, until the spinach or kale is wilted.

Meanwhile, in a large bowl, whisk the eggs. Stir in the hot sauce. Add the egg mixture to the sausage mixture and stir until evenly mixed. Cook without additional stirring for 3 minutes, or until the edges begin to firm. Transfer to the oven and bake for 15 minutes. Allow to cool slightly before serving.

Per serving: 192 calories, 17 g protein, 5 g carbohydrates, 11 g total fat, 4 g saturated fat, 1 g fiber, 644 mg sodium

SPAGHETTI WITH MEATBALLS

This perennial favorite remains a part of your menu simply by replacing conventional pasta with courgette spaghetti and not using bread crumbs in the meatballs.

This recipe is enormously simplified by using one of the spiral cutters discussed earlier in this section to create spaghetti. If you choose to use a store-bought tomato sauce, be sure to choose the brand with the least sugar and, whenever possible, choose brands that use BPA-free cans for tomatoes and tomato purée. Alternatively, make your own sauce from the recipe on the opposite page.

Makes 4 servings

700 g (1½ lb) minced beef

30 g (1 oz) ground golden flaxseeds

1 egg

1 tablespoon chopped fresh basil or
   1 teaspoon dried

1 tablespoon chopped fresh oregano
   or 1 teaspoon dried

1 teaspoon sea salt

1 tablespoon extra-virgin olive oil

1 medium onion, chopped

3–4 cloves garlic, minced

700 g (1½ lb) courgettes, spiral-cut

2 jars (400 g/14 oz) tomato sauce
   or 1 recipe Homemade Tomato
   Sauce (opposite page)

In a medium bowl, combine the beef, flaxseeds, egg, basil, oregano, and salt and mix by hand until thoroughly combined. Form into 2.5 cm (1 in) balls.

In a large frying pan over medium-high heat, heat the oil. Cook the onion and garlic until the onion is translucent. Add the meatballs and cook, turning occasionally to cook all surfaces, for 10 minutes, or until lightly browned on the outside and no longer pink on the inside. Using a slotted spoon, transfer the meatballs and onion mixture to a large serving bowl and cover to keep warm. Add the courgette "spaghetti" to the frying pan and cook, covered, tossing occasionally, for 3 minutes, or until softened but not limp. Serve the spaghetti topped with the meatballs and tomato sauce.

Per serving: 537 calories, 40 g protein, 22 g carbohydrates, 33 g total fat,
11 g saturated fat, 7 g fiber, 1,578 mg sodium

HOMEMADE TOMATO SAUCE

Makes 8 servings

4 tablespoons extra-virgin olive oil, divided

1 small onion, chopped

3 cloves garlic, minced

4 cans (400 g/14 oz each) whole peeled tomatoes

1 can (6 oz) tomato purée

1 teaspoon sea salt

1 tablespoon chopped fresh basil or 1 teaspoon dried

1 tablespoon chopped fresh oregano or 1 teaspoon dried

Ground black pepper to taste

In a large pot over medium-high heat, heat 1 tablespoon of the olive oil. Cook the onion and garlic until the onion is translucent.

Meanwhile, in a blender, blend the tomatoes briefly until smooth.

Transfer the tomatoes to the onion mixture. Add the remaining 3 tablespoons olive oil, the tomato purée, and salt, cover, reduce the heat to medium-low, and simmer for 90 minutes. Stir in the basil, oregano, pepper, and additional salt to taste.

Per serving: 127 calories, 3 g protein, 13 g carbohydrates, 7 g total fat, 1 g saturated fat, 3 g fiber, 788 mg sodium

DAY 5

CURRIED CHICKEN SOUP

Here is a variation on chicken soup that's rich with the flavors of curry, shiitake mushrooms, and coriander. It's thickened with coconut milk to induce satiety. The best results are obtained by using homemade chicken stock, though store-bought (look for brands without wheat flour, cornflour, or other grain derivatives) still yields a delicious end result.

Makes 6 servings

60 ml (2 fl oz) coconut oil

450 g (1 lb) chicken breasts, cubed

110g (4 oz) shiitake mushrooms, sliced

1 litre chicken stock

2 cans (400 ml/14 fl oz) coconut milk

4 tablespoons curry powder

2 tablespoons ground cinnamon

2 tablespoons chopped coriander

¼ teaspoon sea salt

¼ teaspoon ground black pepper

In a large frying pan over medium-high heat, heat the coconut oil. Cook the chicken until lightly browned and no longer pink on the inside. Add the mushrooms and cook, stirring, for 1 to 2 minutes, or until softened.

Stir in the chicken stock and coconut milk. Add the curry powder, cinnamon, coriander, salt, and pepper. Stir until well mixed. Bring to a low simmer to heat through.

Per serving: 463 calories, 20 g protein, 10 g carbohydrates, 41 g total fat, 34 g saturated fat, 5 g fiber, 795 mg sodium

FETTUCCINE ALFREDO

Cheese and butter are among the most benign forms of dairy because of their high fat content and the processes used to create them. However, because this is a dairy-rich dish, you can cut back on your reliance on dairy products, if desired, by replacing the cream with canned coconut milk and the butter with extra-virgin olive oil. Serve with a green vegetable such as steamed green beans or broccoli, or with a salad.

Makes 4 servings

45 g (1½ oz) grated Parmesan cheese

90 g (3 oz) grated Romano or Parmesan cheese

60 g (2½ oz) butter

2 cloves garlic, minced

900 g (2 lb) courgettes, spiral-cut into fettuccine

120 ml (4 fl oz) double cream or canned coconut milk

¼ teaspoon sea salt

Ground black pepper to taste

In a large serving bowl, combine the Parmesan and Romano cheeses and mix. Set aside.

In a large frying pan over medium heat, melt the butter. Cook the garlic, stirring frequently, until it's just fragrant. Add the courgette fettuccine and cook, covered, tossing occasionally, for 3 minutes, or until softened but not wilted. Add the cream or coconut milk and bring to a low simmer, then remove from the heat. Season with the salt and pepper.

Pour the noodle mixture into the bowl with the cheeses, toss, and serve.

Per serving: 368 calories, 13 g protein, 9 g carbohydrates, 31 g total fat, 20 g saturated fat, 2 g fiber, 724 mg sodium

CHOCOLATE AVOCADO PUDDING

Here is a variation on chocolate pudding that is filling and healthy, without the sugar load typical of puddings. The avocados should be ripe so that the pudding is smooth and not bitter. Don't let the small serving size fool you: This pudding will fill you to bursting!

As with many Wheat Belly–style dishes, including goodies like this pudding, because all unhealthy ingredients like sugar and grains have been removed, you can have this pudding for breakfast or lunch as the meal itself. Because the pudding is not heated, it can also serve as a means to obtain prebiotic fibers/resistant starches by incorporating inulin powder, a green banana, or a raw potato. Because avocado is the main ingredient, this pudding is best consumed right away.

Makes 4 servings

3 large ripe avocados, halved and pitted

240 ml (8 fl oz) canned coconut milk

60 g (2½ oz) unsweetened cocoa powder

1 teaspoon vanilla extract

Sweetener equivalent to 115 g (4 oz) sugar

½ teaspoon ground cinnamon

3 tablespoons shredded unsweetened coconut or 110 g (4 oz) fresh berries (optional)

With a spoon, shell the avocado flesh into a blender. Add the coconut milk, cocoa, vanilla, sweetener, and cinnamon and blend until well mixed. Spoon into 4 individual serving bowls and chill in the refrigerator for 30 minutes. Top each serving with coconut or several fresh berries, if using.

Per serving: 342 calories, 6 g protein, 19 g carbohydrates, 32 g total fat, 16 g saturated fat, 12 g fiber, 19 mg sodium

DAY 6

AUBERGINE MINI PIZZAS

Here is an easy way to make a quick and portable single-serving-size pizza that can be handily transported to school or work. Of course, any number of variations are possible by adding different ingredients, such as green peppers, sausage, mushrooms, etc.

Makes 8

1 medium aubergine, sliced crosswise into 1 cm (½ in) thick slices

250 g (9 oz) pizza sauce

50 g (2 oz) sliced pepperoni

35 g (1 oz) shredded mozzarella cheese

3 tablespoons extra-virgin olive oil

Preheat the oven to 190°C/375°F/Gas mark 5.

Arrange the aubergine slices on a baking sheet. Bake for 8 to 10 minutes, or until just lightly browned.

Remove from the oven and spread with the pizza sauce. Place 1 or 2 slices of pepperoni on each aubergine slice, then sprinkle generously with the cheese. Drizzle about 1 teaspoon olive oil over the top of each. Bake for 4 to 5 minutes, or until the cheese is melted.

Per serving: 176 calories, 7 g protein, 11 g carbohydrates, 12 g total fat, 4 g saturated fat, 4 g fiber, 275 mg sodium

PORK THAI STIR-FRY

If you love the flavors of garlic, ginger, curry, and coriander found in many Thai dishes, you'll love this Pork Thai Stir-Fry. This dish can be served alone or, to make it more substantial, served on top of "riced" cauliflower (cauliflower that has been steamed, then pulsed in a food processor or food chopper to reduce it to rice-size granules, as described in the Prawn Fried "Rice" recipe on page 130). Use your choice of pork, such as pork chop, loin, baby back ribs, or ham. All introduce their own unique flavors. Because the fish sauce typically comes quite heavily salted, it's usually not necessary to add additional salt to this dish. Nonetheless, taste your dish before serving to gauge the need for any additional salt.

Makes 4 servings

1 tablespoon coconut oil

2 cloves garlic, minced

4–5 spring onions, chopped

450 g (1 lb) boneless pork or ham, cubed or thinly sliced

1 tablespoon grated fresh ginger

1 large head broccoli, cut into florets

110g (4 oz) shiitake mushrooms, sliced

120 ml (4 fl oz) coconut milk

1 tablespoon red curry sauce

60 ml (2 fl oz) fish sauce

2 tablespoons chopped coriander

In a large frying pan over medium-high heat, heat the coconut oil. Cook the garlic and spring onions until the garlic is fragrant. Add the pork or ham and the ginger. Cook, stirring occasionally, for 7 to 8 minutes, or until the pork is no longer pink.

Add the broccoli, mushrooms, coconut milk, curry sauce, and fish sauce and cook, covered, stirring occasionally, for 5 minutes, or until the broccoli is softened. Top with the coriander before serving.

Per serving: 289 calories, 31 g protein, 11 g carbohydrates, 14 g total fat, 10 g saturated fat, 5 g fiber, 1,565 mg sodium

DAY 7

CHORIZO, PEPPER, AND AVOCADO FRY-UP

We no longer confine breakfast dishes to breakfast, but have them for lunch or dinner, too. Breakfast fry-ups are often exploding with potatoes, but we don't want the blood sugar problems of their excessive starch. We use roasted radishes in place of potatoes. Don't be turned off by the radishes; their taste and texture change substantially with roasting, and they fill out your frying pan just like potatoes with none of the health problems. If you feel it requires too much time and effort to prepare during a busy week, swap this recipe for one of the easier lunch recipes and save this recipe for a weekend lunch when you have more time.

Makes 4 servings

450 g (1 lb) radishes, quartered

4 tablespoons extra-virgin olive oil, divided

½ teaspoon sea salt

½ teaspoon ground black pepper

1 clove garlic, minced

4 spring onions, sliced

350 g (12 oz) chorizo sausage, sliced

1 green pepper, seeded and coarsely sliced

60 g (2½ oz) sliced kale or spinach

4 large eggs

1 large avocado, cut into small cubes

Preheat the oven to 220°C/425°F/Gas mark 7.

In a medium shallow baking pan, combine the radishes, 2 tablespoons of the olive oil, the salt, and black pepper and toss to coat evenly. Roast for 20 minutes. Reduce the heat to 180°C/350°F/Gas mark 4.

Meanwhile, in a cast-iron or other ovenproof frying pan over medium-high heat, heat the remaining 2 tablespoons olive oil. Cook the garlic and spring onions, stirring frequently, for 2 minutes, or until the garlic is fragrant. Add the sausage and pepper and cook, stirring occasionally, until the sausage is no longer pink. Add the kale or spinach, cover, and cook for 2 to 3 minutes, or until wilted. Stir the roasted radishes into the sausage mixture.

With a large spoon, make 4 depressions in the mixture, evenly spaced apart. Crack an egg into each depression. Place in the oven and bake for 10 minutes, or until the eggs set.

Remove from the oven, add additional sea salt and black pepper to taste, and sprinkle the avocado cubes over the top.

Per serving: 689 calories, 30 g protein, 15 g carbohydrates, 57 g total fat, 17 g saturated fat, 6 g fiber, 1,381 mg sodium

BACON-WRAPPED CHICKEN BREASTS STUFFED WITH SPINACH, MUSHROOMS, AND ROASTED RED PEPPERS

Here is a way to have a chicken dish that is nutritionally complete, including plenty of veggies. You might therefore find that just 1 of these stuffed chicken breasts is sufficient as a meal by itself. You can, of course, always add a side dish or salad to suit bigger appetites.

Makes 4 servings

4 boneless, skinless chicken breasts (approximately 900 g/2 lb)

1 tablespoon extra-virgin olive oil

2 cloves garlic, minced

1 medium onion, chopped

110 g (4 oz) portobello mushrooms, sliced

170 g (6 oz) roasted red peppers

120 g (4 oz) fresh spinach or 275 g (10 oz) frozen spinach, thawed and squeezed dry

1 teaspoon sea salt

½ teaspoon ground black pepper

8 rashers bacon (preferably uncured)

Preheat the oven to 180°C/350°F/Gas mark 4.

Lay each chicken breast flat and, with a sharp knife, cut a pocket in each breast by starting at the thickest part and then cutting horizontally, stopping short of cutting all the way through. Set aside.

In a large frying pan over medium-high heat, heat the oil. Cook the garlic and onion for 2 to 3 minutes, or until softened. Add the mushrooms, roasted peppers, spinach, salt, and black pepper and cook, covered, stirring occasionally, for 4 minutes, or until the mushrooms have softened and the spinach is wilted. Transfer to a large bowl and set aside.

Place the chicken breasts in the frying pan and cook for 4 to 6 minutes, turning once, or until both sides are browned. Remove from the heat and place on a large plate. Allow to cool for several minutes, then spoon the reserved spinach mixture into the pocket of each breast and close. Wrap each breast with 2 rashers of bacon in a spiral pattern. Place in a baking dish and bake for 25 minutes, or until the bacon is cooked and a thermometer inserted in the thickest portion of the chicken registers 74°C (165°F).

Per serving: 457 calories, 54 g protein, 6 g carbohydrates, 24 g total fat, 7 g saturated fat, 2 g fiber, 954 mg sodium

DAY 8

SPICY MINESTRONE

Don't you love how the flavors of the vegetables mingle in a good minestrone? Here, we jazz it up a bit further with some peppery hot sauce and basil. Look for BPA-free brands of chopped tomatoes and tomato purée.

Makes 6 servings

4 tablespoons extra-virgin olive oil, divided

1 onion, chopped

2 cloves garlic, minced

1 litre chicken stock

1 litre water

1 can (400 g/14 oz) chopped tomatoes

1 can (175 g/6 oz) tomato purée

2 teaspoons hot-pepper sauce

2 celery sticks, chopped

225 g (8 oz) green beans, cut into 2.5 cm (1 in) pieces

1 can (425 g/15 oz) pinto beans, drained and rinsed

110 g (4 oz) button mushrooms, sliced

1½ teaspoons sea salt

1 teaspoon ground black pepper

120 g (4 oz) chopped fresh spinach or 275 g (10 oz) frozen chopped spinach, thawed and squeezed dry

15 g (½ oz) cup fresh basil, chopped

In a large stockpot over medium-high heat, heat 1 tablespoon of the olive oil. Cook the onion and garlic, stirring frequently, for 2 to 3 minutes, or until softened.

Increase the heat to high and add the stock, water, tomatoes, tomato purée, hot sauce, celery, green beans, pinto beans, mushrooms, remaining 3 tablespoons olive oil, salt, and black pepper. Cover and bring to the boil. Reduce the heat and simmer, partially covered, for 15 minutes. Add the spinach and basil and cook for 10 minutes, or until the vegetables are tender. Taste and adjust the salt and black pepper, if needed.

Per serving: 201 calories, 7 g protein, 22 g carbohydrates, 11 g total fat, 1 g saturated fat, 6 g fiber, 1,583 mg sodium

PRAWN FRIED "RICE"

Absent any grains, this Prawn Fried "Rice," as with many other dishes created for the Wheat Belly lifestyle, is deceptively filling. It can therefore be confidently served by itself for dinner or for another meal.

Makes 4 servings

1 head cauliflower, cut into florets

2 tablespoons coconut oil

5–6 spring onions, chopped

450 g (1 lb) cooked prawns, deveined and tails removed

1 tablespoon grated fresh ginger

155 g (5½ oz) grated carrots

1 green pepper, seeded and chopped

3 tablespoons gluten-free soy sauce or tamari

2 tablespoons fish sauce

2 tablespoons sesame oil

2 eggs

Ground black pepper to taste

Place a steamer basket in a large pot with 5 cm (2 in) of water. Bring to the boil over medium-high heat. Place the cauliflower florets in the basket and steam for 20 minutes, or until softened. Transfer to a food chopper or food processor and pulse to reduce to rice-size pieces.

Meanwhile, in a large frying pan over medium-high heat, heat the coconut oil. Cook the spring onions for 1 to 2 minutes, or until tender. Add the prawns, ginger, carrots, and pepper. Cook, covered, stirring occasionally, for 4 to 5 minutes, or until the carrots and pepper have softened.

Add the riced cauliflower, soy sauce or tamari, fish sauce, sesame oil, eggs, and black pepper and stir until well combined. Cook, covered, stirring occasionally, for 2 minutes, or until the eggs solidify.

Per serving: 347 calories, 32 g protein, 16 g carbohydrates, 18 g total fat, 8 g saturated fat, 5 g fiber, 2,510 mg sodium

DAY 9

JUMBO GINGERBREAD NUT MUFFINS

Once you try these jumbo-size, nut- and oil-rich muffins, you will appreciate how filling they are. They are made with eggs, coconut oil, almonds, and other nuts and seeds, so they are also very healthy. You can also add a schmear of cream cheese or a bit of unsweetened fruit butter for extra flavor. To fill out a lunch, add a chunk of cheese, some fresh berries or sliced fruit, or an avocado. While walnuts and pumpkin seeds are called for in the recipe to add crunch, you can substitute your choice of nut or seed, such as pecans, pistachios, or sunflower seeds.

A jumbo muffin tin is used in this recipe, but a smaller muffin tin can be substituted. If a smaller tin is used, reduce baking time by about 5 minutes, though always assess doneness by inserting a wooden pick into the center of a muffin and making sure it comes out clean. If you make the smaller size, pack 2 muffins for lunch.

Makes 6

60 g (2½ oz) ground almonds/flour

60 g (2½ oz) shredded unsweetened coconut

60 g (2½ oz) chopped walnuts

65 g (2½ oz) pumpkin seeds

Sweetener equivalent to 170 g (6 oz) sugar

2 teaspoons ground cinnamon

1 tablespoon ground ginger

1 teaspoon ground nutmeg

½ teaspoon ground cloves

1 teaspoon sea salt

3 eggs

120 ml (4 fl oz) coconut oil, melted

1 teaspoon vanilla extract

120 ml (4 fl oz) water

Preheat the oven to 180°C/350°F/Gas mark 4.

Place paper liners in a 6-cup jumbo muffin tin or grease the cups with coconut or other oil.

In a large bowl, combine the ground almonds/flour, coconut, walnuts, pumpkin seeds, sweetener, cinnamon, ginger, nutmeg, cloves, and salt. Mix well.

In a medium bowl, whisk the eggs. Stir in the coconut oil, vanilla, and water. Pour the egg mixture into the ground almonds mixture and combine thoroughly.

Divide the batter evenly among the muffin cups. Bake for 30 minutes, or until a wooden pick inserted in the center of a muffin comes out clean.

Per serving (1 muffin): 893 calories, 25 g protein, 26 g carbohydrates, 82 g total fat, 30 g saturated fat, 12 g fiber, 333 mg sodium

BRATWURST WITH PEPPERS
AND SAUERKRAUT

Living in Milwaukee has turned me on to the flavors of German-style bratwurst, but any spicy sausage (such as Italian, chorizo, or a smoked sausage) will do just fine in this recipe. The quality of the brat or sausage makes the dish, so choose your favorite. The spices used in various sausages will vary, so I kept the spices and flavors of the sauerkraut mixture light. However, this makes the choice of bratwurst or sausage the crucial component of this dish. You can also add ground coriander, nutmeg, and other herbs and spices if compatible with your choice of sausage.

Makes 4 servings

1 teaspoon caraway seeds

½ teaspoon celery seeds

2 tablespoons extra-virgin olive oil

450 g (1 lb) bratwurst or other spicy sausages

1 onion, chopped

2 green peppers, seeded and sliced

¼ teaspoon sea salt

Ground black pepper to taste

300 g (11 oz) sauerkraut, drained

Using a mortar and pestle, grind the caraway and celery seeds. Set aside.

In a large frying pan over medium heat, heat the olive oil. Cook the sausages for 15 minutes, or until lightly browned on the outside and barely pink on the inside. (Alternatively, cook on a grill until nearly done.) Add the onion, peppers, reserved caraway and celery seeds, salt, and black pepper. Cover and cook for 5 to 7 minutes, or until the onion is translucent, the peppers are tender, and the sausages are no longer pink.

Add the sauerkraut and toss briefly before serving.

Per serving: 533 calories, 18 g protein, 16 g carbohydrates, 44 g total fat, 15 g saturated fat, 4 g fiber, 1,524 mg sodium

"POTATO" SALAD

To keep with the tradition of having potato salad with bratwurst, here is a way to re-create this dish without incurring the weight-packing effect of potatoes, which are replaced in this recipe with turnips. Before you wrinkle your nose, try it—I predict that you will be surprised. The only hurdle you might encounter is the bitterness that some people perceive with turnips. To minimize the bitter effect, use salt a bit more liberally and choose smaller turnips.

Makes 4 servings

4 litres water

2 teaspoons sea salt

900 g (2 lb) turnips, stems and roots removed

250 g (9 oz) mayonnaise

½ white onion, chopped

2 medium dill pickles, chopped

2 teaspoons Dijon mustard

2 tablespoons white vinegar

1 teaspoon ground paprika

½ teaspoon ground black pepper

2 eggs, hard-boiled and sliced

½ teaspoon sea salt

In a large pot, bring the water and salt to a boil.

Meanwhile, chop the turnips into approximately 2.5 cm (1 in) pieces. Add to the boiling water, cover, and cook for 8 to 10 minutes, or until tender. Drain. Allow to cool for 5 minutes, or run under cold running water briefly and drain.

In a large bowl, combine the turnips, mayonnaise, onion, pickles, mustard, vinegar, paprika, pepper, eggs, and salt. Mix well and serve.

Per serving: 492 calories, 5 g protein, 13 g carbohydrates, 47 g total fat, 7 g saturated fat, 4 g fiber, 1,130 mg sodium

DAY 10

BLT WRAP

Here is a way to enjoy a wrap filled with your favorite ingredients. In this simple recipe, we fill the wrap with perennial favorites bacon, lettuce, and tomato. This recipe works best as a weekend lunch at home, rather than a lunch consumed at work or school, since this BLT Wrap should be assembled just before consuming or it will become soggy.

The key with making the flaxseed wrap is cooking time: undercooked and it will be runny; overcooked and it will be too stiff to wrap around the fillings. In the microwave, the amount of time that was just right for me was 90 seconds, or 8 minutes in the oven at 180°C/350°F/Gas mark 4. You may have to modify your cooking time slightly to accommodate your microwave. But once you get the hang of it, you will be rewarded with a delicious, sturdy wrap.

It's not a BLT without mayonnaise, so choose your mayonnaise carefully and make sure it does not contain wheat flour, cornflour, or other grain ingredients. If it is made with less-than-perfect oils, such as soya or safflower, the small quantity required should not be a concern.

Makes 1

30 g (1 oz) ground golden flaxseeds	1 tablespoon water
½ teaspoon onion powder	1 tablespoon mayonnaise
Generous dash of sea salt	20 g (¾ oz) lettuce or spinach leaves
1 egg	2 rashers bacon, cooked
1½ tablespoons extra-virgin olive oil or coconut oil, melted	1 slice tomato, quartered

Generously grease a 23 cm (9 in) microwaveable or ovenproof pie plate and set aside.

In a small bowl, combine the flaxseeds, onion powder, and salt. Mix well. Stir in the egg, oil, and water and combine thoroughly. The consistency should be that of a thick but pourable liquid. If it's too thick, add a teaspoon of water and mix.

Pour the mixture into the pie plate and tilt and rotate to cover the entire bottom, or use a spoon to spread. Microwave on high power for 90 seconds. (Cooking time may vary depending on your microwave oven; adjust as needed.) Alternatively, cook the mixture on the hob in a greased 25 cm (10 in) frying pan over medium-low heat for 2½ to 3 minutes. Turn the wrap and cook the other side for 30 seconds.

Allow to cool for 2 minutes. Using a spatula, lift the edges carefully and transfer the wrap to a plate, rough side up.

With a spoon, spread a stripe of mayonnaise down the center of the wrap. Arrange the lettuce or spinach, bacon, and tomato along the stripe, then roll.

Per serving: 580 calories, 19 g protein, 11 g carbohydrates, 53 g total fat, 8 g saturated fat, 9 g fiber, 637 mg sodium

ROASTED BRUSSELS SPROUTS AND HAM FRY-UP

Here is another example of having breakfast for dinner. (The opposite concept—dinner for breakfast—works equally well in this lifestyle.) After all, we have turned the traditional notion of a grain-based breakfast inside out, breaking all the former "rules" of what is for breakfast and what is for dinner.

I snuck a sweet potato into this recipe for a bit of beta-carotene and flavor; it adds only 5 grams net carbs per serving. The eggs are optional in this recipe, in case you don't want to take the breakfast-for-dinner idea all the way through.

Makes 4 servings

2 tablespoons extra-virgin olive oil or coconut oil

2 cloves garlic, minced

1 onion, chopped

450 g (1 lb) Brussels sprouts, halved

110 g (4 oz) portobello mushrooms, sliced

1 medium sweet potato, cut into 1 cm (½ in) cubes

1 teaspoon sea salt

350 g (12 oz) ham, cubed

4 eggs (optional)

25 g (1 oz) grated Parmesan cheese (optional)

Preheat the oven to 180°C/350°F/Gas mark 4.

In a large ovenproof frying pan over medium-high heat, heat the oil. Cook the garlic and onion for 2 minutes, or until the onion is translucent. Add the Brussels sprouts, mushrooms, sweet potato, and salt and stir. Cook, covered, stirring occasionally, for 7 to 8 minutes, or until the Brussels sprouts and mushrooms soften. Stir in the ham.

If desired, use a spoon to form 4 small evenly spaced depressions in the mixture. Crack an egg into each. Sprinkle the cheese over the top, if using.

Transfer the frying pan to the oven and bake for 10 minutes.

Per serving: 247 calories, 19 g protein, 20 g carbohydrates, 11 g total fat, 3 g saturated fat, 6 g fiber, 929 mg sodium

CHAPTER 6

WHEAT BELLY 10-DAY DETOX SECRET SAUCE

Fat Blasters, Snacks, and Healthy Waters

MOM LIKELY HAD a secret sauce. Grandma had a secret sauce, maintaining a curious silence when pressed for the recipe. Even fast-food restaurants have a secret sauce.

Well, here is *your* secret sauce—several additional strategies that further compound your success in navigating the week and a half of the Wheat Belly 10-Day Detox. None of these are truly "secret," but they are unusual and uncommon, yielding a number of unique advantages in your detox process, even beyond the considerable benefits obtained with the nutritional supplement and prebiotic fiber strategies discussed earlier. The Wheat Belly Detox Secret Sauce strategies compound the benefits of this lifestyle, while also providing a way to obtain some of the nutrients recommended in previous chapters. They can be consumed during the 10 days of your detox program or anytime afterward. You can make a limited supply to suit your own purposes, or you can whip up larger batches so that they can be shared with everyone in the family.

In this chapter, you will find recipes for Fat Blasters, simple snacks packed with satiating fats that can come to your rescue whenever cravings strike during your detox process. If hunger or cravings overcome you during the detox—or at any other time, for that matter—*always* consider inadequate fat intake; Fat Blasters are a quick, convenient, and tasty way to remedy your lack of fat. There are also recipes for portable snack balls that are safe for consumption during your 10-day detox and will not disrupt

---

JOAN, 50, travel agent, New York

"I *love* pasta, rice, and grains. I could live on those and veggies. I'm not a big meat eater, so giving up grains was giving up a *major* part of my diet.

"I began the detox feeling tired, headachy, lethargic, not myself. I had to take Advil to get rid of the headaches; they wouldn't go away on their own. After 2 days, I felt a lot better. I have had a feeling of peace. I have felt calmer.

"I'm not hungry anymore; I'm eating healthy food and feeling completely satisfied. My cravings for food have gone away—big time. As Dr. Davis mentioned, you can sometimes go a long time without eating. I had become a big sweets eater over the years, and, incredibly, by eating grain-free, I've noticed that my cravings have gone away. I have to admit, I didn't think that could happen to me.

"Sleep: There has been a pretty big change here. I have been dreaming just about every night, like when I was a kid. I think that means I am getting a deeper sleep than I was previously.

"The detox takes a lot of planning, a lot of shopping, and a lot of cleaning up, so I think you have to be organized. You have to get yourself prepared on the weekend for the week ahead."

By the end of her detox experience, Joan had lost 5.2 pounds, or 3.4 percent of her starting body weight.

weight loss or health efforts. Eat as many Fat Blasters or detox snacks as you like. Remember: We do *not* worry about calories or portion sizes in the Wheat Belly lifestyle. (You will quickly discover how filling these snacks are, and eating even two or three can be a challenge.)

There is also a simple recipe for Coconut Magnesium Water that you can use as a convenient and surprisingly effective way to obtain magnesium to prevent or relieve muscle cramps and gain faster relief from health issues such as migraine headaches, high blood pressure, and even heart rhythm disorders. There is also a simple recipe for Coconut Electrolyte Replacement Water that can be used to replace electrolytes, such as potassium and magnesium, without the expense of the electrolyte waters sold in stores. Lastly, I provide some creative ways to liven up your drinking water to ensure that you are taking in sufficient fluids and sodium, which is especially important during the withdrawal process of your detox.

WHEAT BELLY DETOX FAT BLASTERS

Fat Blasters are bite-size wallops of healthy fat that give you a feeling of fullness without triggering insulin—the hormone of weight gain—thereby allowing weight loss to proceed unimpeded, or even accelerating the process. Fat Blasters are high in calories and high in fat grams—and that's *good*.

Fat Blasters can be eaten as a snack, or you can eat two or three (or more) as a meal replacement. (In general, of course, you should be sure to have real, whole foods for most meals to ensure full nutrient intake. Fat Blasters are meant to be an occasional component of your diet.) Fat Blasters can be especially useful when you are in the process of losing weight and want to reverse the metabolic distortions of a wheat belly, especially visceral fat, high blood sugars, and fatty liver, the accumulation of fat in the liver that accompanies visceral fat. (Remember: It's not fat that causes fat accumulation in the liver; it's sugar and the amylopectin A of grains.) Fat Blasters can help push you closer to the power of ketosis, the natural physiologic process that develops in response to carbohydrate elimination that accelerates weight loss and helps reverse many health conditions. Achieving metabolic ketosis is *not* necessary to succeed in the Wheat Belly 10-Day Detox, but it is an optional means of accelerating your success. Contrary to popular opinion, achieving ketosis does not require greater protein intake; it requires greater *fat* intake while maintaining near zero intake of carbohydrates. Wheat Belly Detox Fat Blasters can be used to take you a step or two closer to this effect.

Note that, because the melting point of coconut oil is 24°C (76°F), these goodies are best stored in the refrigerator; otherwise, you will have a gooey mess at room temperature. (This is one of the reasons that food manufacturers will hydrogenate coconut oil to keep foods solid at room temperature, but we don't want any hydrogenated or trans fats in our diet.)

Because we live in an era in which most people have been misled by fat phobia, it is often tough to get all the fat we need when eating outside the home. Meats will often be served lean, for instance, with the fat removed. To be sure you get the fat you need to succeed in this lifestyle, you can carry Fat Blasters with you in small containers. If stored at cooler temperatures below the melting point, they will remain solid. If carried at higher temperatures, however, you will have to drink your Fat Blaster. It will taste the same, and the health and satiety effects still apply, but be sure to choose sealable containers that won't leak should the oil liquefy.

For ease of removal and cleanup, use paper or silicone cupcake liners placed in mini muffin tins. Standard muffin tins also work just fine, though you will end up with a smaller number of larger Blasters with these recipes. If you don't have a muffin tin, you can use an ice cube tray.

Because Fat Blasters are nearly pure oil, it is best to choose liquid sweeteners, such as pure liquid stevia or monk fruit. Dry sweeteners do not dissolve easily in oil. If your sweetener comes in crystalline form, pulse a batch of sweetener in a food chopper or food processor to reduce it to the consistency of confectioners' sugar; this will prevent the crystals from yielding an undesirable crunchy effect.

PEANUT BUTTER CUP FAT BLASTERS

Does it get much better than this? You will get better results if you refrigerate the peanut butter for at least 1 hour prior to using it. The stiffer texture will allow it to remain between the chocolate layers and not disperse into the mix.

Makes 20

225 g (8 oz) unsweetened chocolate (100% cacao), broken into pieces

240 ml (8 fl oz) coconut oil, melted

Sweetener equivalent to 115 g (4 oz) sugar

125 g (4½ oz) unsweetened natural peanut butter, chilled

80 g (3 oz) finely chopped dry-roasted peanuts, walnuts, or pecans (optional)

Place paper liners in 20 cups of a mini muffin tin.

In a microwaveable bowl, microwave the chocolate on high power in 20-second increments, stirring after each interval, until melted. Alternatively, melt the chocolate in a double boiler. Add the coconut oil and sweetener and mix thoroughly.

Spoon 1 teaspoon of the mixture into each lined cup, tilting the pan to coat the sides. Place the muffin tin in the freezer for 10 minutes.

Remove the muffin tin from the freezer. Spoon approximately 1 teaspoon of the chilled peanut butter into the center of each cup. Divide the remaining chocolate mixture evenly among the cups, covering the peanut butter. Sprinkle the nuts over the top of each, if using.

Refrigerate for at least 1 hour before eating, or place in the freezer for 30 minutes.

Store in the refrigerator.

Per serving (1 blaster): 195 calories, 3 g protein, 5 g carbohydrates, 21 g total fat, 14 g saturated fat, 2 g fiber, 25 mg sodium

Per serving (1 blaster with optional peanuts): 216 calories, 4 g protein, 5 g carbohydrates, 22 g total fat, 14 g saturated fat, 3 g fiber, 25 mg sodium

RASPBERRY CHEESECAKE FAT BLASTERS

You'll think you've died and gone to heaven with these little morsels of cheese-cake. You can easily substitute any berry, such as strawberries or blueberries, for the raspberries.

Makes 20

225 g (8 oz) organic cream cheese, at room temperature

180 ml (6 fl oz) coconut oil, melted

60 g (2½ oz) raspberries

Sweetener equivalent to 115 g (4 oz) sugar

1 teaspoon vanilla extract

Place paper liners in 20 cups of a mini muffin tin.

In a large bowl, using an electric mixer, blend the cream cheese, coconut oil, raspberries, sweetener, and vanilla until thoroughly combined.

Evenly divide the mixture among the lined cups and refrigerate for at least 1 hour before eating, or place in the freezer for 30 minutes.

Store in the refrigerator.

Per serving (1 blaster): 114 calories, 1 g protein, 1 g carbohydrates, 12 g total fat, 9 g saturated fat, 0 g fiber, 36 mg sodium

ORANGE CREAM FAT BLASTERS

While this version features orange and is meant to mimic the flavor of an orange Creamsicle, you can easily substitute lemon extract and lemon peel for a lemony variation.

Makes 20

225 g (8 oz) organic cream cheese, at room temperature

120 ml (4 fl oz) coconut oil, melted

1 tablespoon orange extract

1 tablespoon orange peel

Sweetener equivalent to 115 g (4 oz) sugar

Place paper liners in 20 cups of a mini muffin tin.

In a large bowl, using an electric mixer, blend the cream cheese, coconut oil, orange extract, orange peel, and sweetener until thoroughly combined.

Evenly divide the mixture among the lined cups and refrigerate for at least 1 hour before eating, or place in the freezer for 30 minutes.

Store in the refrigerator.

Per serving (1 blaster): 88 calories, 1 g protein, 1 g carbohydrates, 9 g total fat, 7 g saturated fat, 0 g fiber, 36 mg sodium

CHOCOLATE COCONUT FAT BLASTERS

Makes 20

225 g (8 oz) unsweetened chocolate (100% cacao), broken into pieces

120 ml (4 fl oz) + 1 tablespoon coconut oil, melted, divided

Sweetener equivalent to 115 g (4 oz) cup sugar

30 g (1 oz) shredded unsweetened coconut

20 whole dry-roasted almonds

Place paper liners in 20 cups of a mini muffin tin.

In a microwaveable bowl, microwave the chocolate on high power in 20-second increments, stirring after each interval, until melted. Alternatively, melt the chocolate in a double boiler. Stir in the 120 ml (4 fl oz) of the coconut oil and the sweetener and mix thoroughly.

Spoon 1 teaspoon of the mixture into each lined cup, tilting the pan to coat the sides. Place the muffin tin in the freezer for 10 minutes.

Meanwhile, in a small bowl, combine the coconut and remaining 1 tablespoon coconut oil. Mix together.

Remove the muffin tin from the freezer. Spoon about 1 teaspoon of the shredded coconut mixture into each cup, then place 1 almond on top of each. Divide the remaining chocolate mixture evenly among the cups, covering the shredded coconut and almond.

Refrigerate for at least 1 hour before eating, or place in the freezer for 30 minutes.

Store in the refrigerator.

Per serving (1 blaster): 137 calories, 2 g protein, 4 g carbohydrates, 15 g total fat, 11 g saturated fat, 2 g fiber, 2 mg sodium

WHEAT BELLY DETOX
SNACK BALLS

Here are healthy Snack Ball recipes that fit into your detox process. Snack Balls are compact packets of calories and fat—because we don't limit either—that are easy to carry and portable. They're also tasty and filling and thereby serve as useful snacks.

Having an arsenal of healthy snacks can be important because it gives you healthy options to turn to instead of the unhealthy snacks that can booby-trap your detox program while you're at work or school, traveling, or in other situations where healthy food is unavailable. These Snack Balls fit easily into your 10-day detox to consume as you like, but be warned: They are exceptionally filling. (You'll find additional safe goodies in the next chapter.)

As part of our effort to cultivate bowel flora species diversity for improved overall health, I included inulin powder in each of these recipes sufficient to provide approximately 1 gram of prebiotic fibers/resistant starch per ball. Feel free to increase the inulin or fructooligosaccharide (FOS), especially as you get deeper into the detox program and onward, as a convenient means of obtaining your daily dose of prebiotic fibers. The inulin and FOS are optional, however, and can be included or excluded without affecting the recipe.

With any of these snacks, taste your dough before rolling it into balls and adjust the sweetener to taste. Remember that your sense of sweetness is going to change the further into your detox you go, so you will need less sweetener as time passes.

TRAIL MIX BALLS

Here are bite-size morsels of fat, protein, fiber, and flavor that will satisfy any wild sweet-tooth impulse that breaks through, especially during your first week of the detox process. Like all Wheat Belly recipes, however, these Trail Mix Balls are also healthy choices for situations outside of your detox experience and can therefore serve as a healthy snack for just about any situation. The use of refrigerated almond butter makes forming the balls easier.

Makes 20

130 g (4½ oz) raw pumpkin seeds

100 g (3½ oz) pecans

60 g (2½ oz) shredded unsweetened coconut

30 g (1 oz) raisins

1 teaspoon ground cinnamon

1 tablespoon inulin or FOS powder

Sweetener equivalent to 55 g (2 oz) sugar

240 g (8 oz) almond butter, chilled

In a food chopper or processor, combine the pumpkin seeds, pecans, coconut, and raisins. Pulse until reduced to granules. Transfer to a large bowl.

Add the cinnamon, inulin or FOS, and sweetener and mix thoroughly. Stir in the almond butter until completely mixed. Divide the dough into twenty 2.5 cm (1 in) balls. Store in the refrigerator.

Per serving (1 ball): 201 calories, 6 g protein, 7 g carbohydrates, 18 g total fat, 4 g saturated fat, 3 g fiber, 31 mg sodium

COCONUT SNACK BALLS

Because it's full of healthy fat and potassium, coconut figures prominently in the Wheat Belly lifestyle. These little balls make the best of coconut-based ingredients and turn them into bite-size snacks.

Makes 20

100 g (3½ oz) pecans

125 g (4½ oz) raw sunflower seeds

90 g (3 oz) shredded unsweetened coconut, divided

Sweetener equivalent to 2 tablespoons sugar

1 tablespoon inulin or FOS powder

240 g (8 oz) almond butter, chilled

60 ml (2 fl oz) coconut oil, melted

1 teaspoon vanilla extract

1 teaspoon natural coconut extract

In a food chopper or processor, combine the pecans, sunflower seeds, and two-thirds of the coconut. Pulse until reduced to granules. Transfer to a large bowl.

On a medium plate, pour the remaining coconut and spread evenly. Set aside.

Add the sweetener, inulin or FOS, almond butter, coconut oil, vanilla, and coconut extract to the pecan mixture and mix thoroughly. Divide the dough into twenty 2.5 cm (1 in) balls and roll each ball in the coconut on the plate. Refrigerate for at least 1 hour before serving. Store in the refrigerator.

Per serving (1 ball): 218 calories, 5 g protein, 7 g carbohydrates, 20 g total fat, 7 g saturated fat, 4 g fiber, 3 mg sodium

PB&J SANDWICH BALLS

These balls taste like mini peanut butter and jelly sandwiches that you can just pop in your mouth as a healthy snack. Because of the natural sweetness of the strawberries and peanut butter, the use of a sweetener is optional.

Makes 20

25 g (1 oz) freeze-dried strawberries

1 cup walnuts

130 g (4½ oz) raw pumpkin seeds

30 g (1 oz) shredded unsweetened coconut

185 g (6 oz) unsweetened natural peanut butter, chilled

120 g (4 oz) dry-roasted peanuts, chopped

1 tablespoon inulin or FOS powder

Sweetener equivalent to 2 teaspoons sugar (optional)

In a food chopper or processor, combine the strawberries, walnuts, pumpkin seeds, and coconut. Pulse until reduced to granules. Transfer to a large bowl.

Add the peanut butter, peanuts, inulin or FOS, and sweetener (if using) and stir until thoroughly mixed. Form into twenty 2.5 cm (1 in) balls. Refrigerate for at least 1 hour before serving. Store in the refrigerator.

Per serving (1 ball): 206 calories, 7 g protein, 9 g carbohydrates, 17 g total fat, 3 g saturated fat, 3 g fiber, 3 mg sodium

MAGNESIUM WATER, ELECTROLYTE REPLACEMENT WATER, AND FLAVORED WATERS

Here are two very easy ways to obtain healthy magnesium in a highly absorbable form and electrolytes when needed, such as with strenuous exercise, excessive sweating, or a diarrheal illness. These waters are also inexpensive, saving money over the considerable expense of store-bought magnesium supplements and electrolyte drinks.

COCONUT MAGNESIUM WATER

This simple recipe shows you how to make a healthy coconut water rich in magnesium bicarbonate, the most highly absorbable form of magnesium that effectively restores magnesium in the body while yielding the least potential for diarrhea (since most magnesium supplements are plagued by a laxative effect, causing even more magnesium lost with the diarrhea—not a good strategy). Use Coconut Magnesium Water *in place of magnesium supplements* (don't take both) to avoid long-term magnesium overload.

A 120 ml (4 fl oz) serving of Coconut Magnesium Water provides 90 milligrams of elemental magnesium; 120 ml (4 fl oz) twice per day thereby adds an additional 180 milligrams of elemental magnesium to your daily intake. You can drink up to 450 ml (16 fl oz) per day, which provides a total of 360 milligrams of magnesium per day, which is especially useful during the 10 days of your detox to rapidly restore magnesium.

I find this Coconut Magnesium Water yields an advantage over magnesium in tablet or capsule form. The magnesium bicarbonate from this water is better absorbed and yields better and faster relief from muscle cramps and migraine headaches, and even abnormal heart rhythms—benefits that are more likely to occur with the higher 360 milligrams per day dose.

Note that the milk of magnesia used in the recipe *must* be unflavored, as flavorings block the reaction creating the magnesium bicarbonate. Be sure to label your bottle of Coconut Magnesium Water to prevent any unexpected guzzling by someone unaware that it is magnesium water (which can result in diarrhea). Magnesium water does not need to be refrigerated if consumed within 1 week.

The recipe as written suggests adding coconut extract for a light coconut flavor, but you can substitute any natural extract, such as orange, lemon, or berry. If light sweetness is desired, you can use one of the flavored stevias available in place of the coconut extract; I used 20 drops of berry-flavored SweetLeaf Sweet Drops that yielded a light and pleasant sweetness, subtle enough to allow sipping over ice without being overly sweet.

Makes 8 servings or 16 servings

1 bottle (2 litres) soda water

3 tablespoons unflavored milk of
  magnesia

1 tablespoon coconut extract

Uncap the soda water and pour off a few tablespoons. Shake the milk of magnesia, then pour out 3 tablespoons. (Most brands come with a handy little measuring cup that works perfectly.) Slowly pour the milk of magnesia into the soda water, followed by the coconut extract.

Cap the bottle securely, then shake until all of the sediment has dissolved. Allow to sit for 15 minutes to clarify. If any sediment remains, shake again. Drink 110 ml (4 fl oz) to 225 ml (8 fl oz) twice per day.

COCONUT ELECTROLYTE
REPLACEMENT WATER

The Coconut Magnesium Water (page 150), while a terrific option to supplement magnesium, is intended only as a way to obtain magnesium; it does not replace electrolytes such as potassium and sodium lost during strenuous exercise, summer-time sweating, or a diarrheal illness, or through the fluid loss that develops with the wheat and grain withdrawal process. Here is a way to take advantage of the Coconut Magnesium Water you've made and use it as the basis for an electrolyte-rich but sippable water that you can use to rehydrate and replenish electrolytes. Additional sweetness or flavor can be obtained with stevia and/or flavored stevia drops.

We use conventional coconut water as a source of potassium; it is important to choose an unsweetened brand to minimize sugar. The bicarbonate of soda provides a means of alkalinizing this solution, helping to counteract the excessive acidity that can contribute to many health conditions.

Drink this electrolyte-rich water just as you would any other water.

Makes 5 servings (5 cups)

1 litre water

120 ml (4 fl oz) Coconut Magnesium
  Water (page 150)

120 ml (4 fl oz) unsweetened coconut
  water

½ teaspoon bircarbonate soda

In a large bottle, combine the water, Coconut Magnesium Water, coconut water, and bicarbonate of soda. Shake well. Store in the refrigerator.

Per serving: 4 calories, 0 g protein, 1 g carbohydrates, 0 g total fat, 0 g saturated fat, 0 g fiber, 158 mg sodium

HERB- AND FRUIT-FLAVORED DRINKING WATERS

Every so often, as I steer people back to making plain water their dominant fluid intake, someone will say, "But I can't stand plain water!" Well, first recognize that this, like the desire for excessive sweetness, may be a wheat/grain-induced perception that may disappear along with the grains. But, if your aversion to plain water persists and you don't find enough variety in teas, infusions ("teas" made from herbs, dried fruit, spices, or flowers), and coffee, try making your own herb- and fruit-flavored waters. Recall that the process of wheat and grain withdrawal can involve loss of water and reversal of inflammation that can lead to dehydration. Therefore, it's important to increase our intake of fluids, as well as sodium, during the detox process. This is why a modest quantity of sodium is added to our waters as sodium bicarbonate, or baking soda.

Start with either plain (filtered, spring, or distilled) water or Coconut Electrolyte Replacement Water (see opposite page). In a 2-litre or larger pitcher or a glass water dispenser you keep on your counter, add 1 teaspoon bicarbonate of soda per litre of water if starting with plain water. (Skip the bicarbonate of soda if you're starting with Coconut Electrolyte Replacement Water.) Then add:

Lemon Ginger Water: half of a thinly sliced lemon and 1 tablespoon coarsely grated fresh ginger

Cucumber Lime Water: one-quarter of a thinly sliced cucumber and half of a thinly sliced lime

Strawberry Mint Water: 3 to 4 large thinly sliced strawberries and 6 to 8 fresh mint leaves

Adjust the quantity of herbs and fruit to suit the size of your pitcher or dispenser; the quantities listed above will be sufficient for 2 litres of water.

You get the idea. Other flavor possibilities include halved and sliced oranges, quartered and sliced grapefruit, sliced kiwifruit, peach wedges, or fresh basil. If you'd prefer a bit of sweetness, place the fruit in the bottom of the pitcher first, mash lightly to express the juice, and then add the water. Alternatively, you can add a few drops of plain or flavored stevia or liquid monk fruit.

Another variation is to start with a sun tea, which is a tea brewed over several hours of sitting in bright sunlight. (Choose a clear glass container covered with a lid to keep out pests.) Sun tea can be drunk as is over ice or used as the base for one of the herb- or fruit-flavored waters above. Specialty tea shops now sell an astounding variety of delicious flavors that can be brewed as regular tea or sun tea, but using them as the base for herb- and fruit-flavored waters really opens up endless possibilities to suit your personal tastes.

THE WHEAT BELLY
FAMILY DETOX

Secret Weapons to Convert
Your Family to This Lifestyle

LET'S FACE IT: You may discover levels of health and weight loss that you previously thought unattainable, effortlessly slipping into a new size 8 dress or the old pair of jeans you thought would never fit again, or just feeling and looking better and younger than you have in years . . . but your spouse and family may blow this all off as just another rant, fad, or too much trouble to follow your lead. After all, you're threatening to take away their beloved pizza, pretzels, and beer.

The many thousands of people who have shared their experiences with me and encountered up-front resistance from others report that all it often takes to create believers is for your spouse and family to observe *your* health and weight transformation, your newly found calm and great mood, clear skin, youthfulness, and slenderness, and they will be convinced that they should follow your example and embrace this lifestyle as well. After all, by following this lifestyle, husbands can lose their bellies and man breasts, rediscover youthful energy, and reverse erectile dysfunction, while kids can increase their attention spans and get better grades, experience freedom from bellyaches and emotional excesses, and reduce or eliminate teenage acne.

But sometimes it takes *more* than that to persuade your spouse and kids that this lifestyle puts them back in control of their appetite, health, and weight without depriving them of familiar foods. As with the hard-hitting, rapid-fire 10-Day Menu Plan in this book, these "Secret Weapons" are new to the Wheat Belly program, fresh and ready to be unbundled and used to your advantage.

The recipes for the Secret Weapons provided in this chapter therefore can be used to help convert your family to this lifestyle. These Secret Weapons don't take the form of threatened physical violence or passive-aggressive withholding of favors, but instead are irresistible wheat- and grain-free recipes for foods such as

---

JENNIFER, 48, homemaker, Connecticut

"I felt great for the first 3 or 4 days. I thought I was going to be one of the lucky ones who escapes all symptoms. But then, for the next 3 days, I felt like I got hit by a truck. Really low energy, headaches and fogginess, and irritability. It was ugly and I was discouraged. About midway through Day 8, it all lifted and I felt great—energized, focused, ready to go. It was worth waiting for!

"To relieve my headaches, I took over-the-counter pain relievers. Other than that, I tried to get plenty of rest and drank a ton of water.

"My husband has noticed that I've lost weight, and when I was out with some girlfriends, they told me my skin looked great. I didn't have any makeup on, and they were unaware of my detox, so that was nice!"

Jennifer lost 7.8 pounds with her detox experience, along with an impressive 6.25 total inches lost off her measurements.

Deep-Dish Pepperoni Pizza, Peanut Butter Cookies, and other great persuaders, all created to be safe and consistent with this lifestyle. All of these recipes are also safe for you to include during or after your 10-day detox experience since they are consistent with the Wheat Belly lifestyle. You can, for instance, use any of the dishes in our Secret Weapon arsenal as a substitute for any of the dishes in the 10-Day Menu Plan (except for Detox Shakes, which provide prebiotic fibers).

WHEAT BELLY: GREAT PERSUADERS

Many people do not want to engage in this lifestyle if they (1) do not appreciate the magnitude of health benefits that develop, (2) believe that food will become dull and tasteless and that many former indulgences will be banished, and (3) fear that, by following this lifestyle, their entire lives will become boring, colorless failures with all their friends vacating the scene.

You now understand that the elimination of wheat and grains is unmatched in its potential to help children as well as adults regain health and normal weight, while also the furthest thing from dull. Recall that, minus the taste-distorting effect of wheat and grains, foods actually *taste better* than they did before you undertook your detox, a reflection of the tongue-to-colon recovery of gastrointestinal health. It's not uncommon, for instance, for kids who formerly hated broccoli or Brussels sprouts to begin *loving* them.

Despite your epiphany, you may be encountering the skeptical looks of family who have watched you attempt (and fail) other diets and fads in the past, and who dismiss this as just another passing whim that you will soon fail at and forget. So maybe you don't even tell the family that they are eating wheat- and grain-free. (They may have observed your frantic clearing of the cupboards and refrigerator of all things wheat and grains, but they may not appreciate that a specific dish conforms to your new lifestyle.) Just serve these unique dishes and let them tell you how terrific they smell and taste and how satisfying they are. Tell them to eat more pizza and cheesecake, *then* reveal your secret!

Following are a handful of recipes for what I call the Great Persuaders, or what you and I might secretly call the Great Grain Dissuaders, since after just one taste, the eater will understand that deprivation is not a requirement to enjoy the benefits of this lifestyle. Some are sweet, others are savory: Choose the ones that you believe will pack the greatest punch at those Wheat Bellies in the family—during the 10-day detox and beyond.

BUFFALO CHICKEN WINGS

Is the path to the heart paved in game-time goodies? Maybe so, so here is an option to help please those engaged in Saturday Night Football while staying true to your wheat- and grain-free lifestyle.

Be sure to choose a safe mayonnaise for the blue cheese dressing, one free of wheat flour and cornflour, as well as other unhealthy additives. As a time-saver, you can purchase a blue cheese dressing that doesn't contain any undesirable ingredients.

Makes about 6 servings (4 wings each)

WINGS

125 g (4½ oz) butter, melted

9 tablespoons hot-pepper sauce

2 tablespoons white or apple cider vinegar

1 teaspoon sea salt

1.35 kg (3 lb) chicken wings

BLUE CHEESE DRESSING

250 g (9 oz) mayonnaise

115 g (4 oz) crumbled blue cheese

250 g (9 oz) sour cream

½ teaspoon sea salt

Celery and/or carrot sticks (optional)

To make the wings: In a small bowl, combine the butter, hot sauce, vinegar, and salt. Mix well. Reserve 3–4 tablespoons and set aside. Pour the remaining marinade into a large bowl. Add the wings and toss to coat with the marinade. Marinate in the refrigerator for 60 minutes, turning occasionally.

To make the dressing: Meanwhile, in a small bowl, combine the mayonnaise, blue cheese, sour cream, and salt. Mix well. Refrigerate until serving.

Place an oven rack approximately 20 cm (8 in) from the grill. Preheat the grill. Cover a rimmed baking sheet with foil. Arrange the wings on the baking sheet with space between each wing. Grill for 14 to 16 minutes, turning once, or until the wings are crispy. Watch the wings closely to avoid burning.

Transfer the wings to a serving plate and spread the reserved hot sauce mixture over the top. Serve with the blue cheese dressing and celery and/or carrot sticks, if using.

Per serving: 893 calories, 42 g protein, 2 g carbohydrates, 79 g total fat, 24 g saturated fat, 0 g fiber, 1,301 mg sodium

CHICAGO-STYLE DEEP-DISH PEPPERONI PIZZA

Here's a real winner in the Wheat Belly lifestyle—a thick, luscious Chicago-style pizza that is virtually guaranteed to wow the family.

Even more than with conventional pizza crusts, it is important to use a thick pizza sauce to minimize water that can otherwise yield a soggy crust. If your sauce is too thin, simmer it over low heat for at least 30 minutes, stirring occasionally, to remove the excess moisture.

We use a cast-iron or other ovenproof frying pan in this recipe, but a deep-dish pizza pan works well, too.

Makes 4 servings

200 g (7 oz) ground almonds/flour

½ teaspoon sea salt

1 teaspoon dried basil

2 teaspoons dried oregano

150 g (5 oz) shredded mozzarella cheese, divided

2 eggs

120 ml (4 fl oz) extra-virgin olive oil, divided

60 ml (2 fl oz) water

1 small onion, finely chopped

1 small pepper, chopped

400 g (14 oz) pizza sauce

110 g (4 oz) pepperoni, sliced

Preheat the oven to 190°C/375°F/Gas mark 5.

In a medium bowl, combine the ground almonds/flour, salt, basil, oregano, and half of the cheese. In a small bowl, whisk the eggs with 2 tablespoons of the olive oil. Stir in the water.

Pour the egg mixture into the ground almonds/flour mixture and mix thoroughly. Set aside.

In a 25.5 cm (10 in) diameter cast-iron or other ovenproof frying pan over medium-high heat, heat 1 tablespoon of the olive oil. Cook the onion and pepper for 3 minutes, or until the onion is translucent. Remove from the heat and transfer the onion mixture to a bowl. Pour off and discard any liquid from the bowl.

Allow the frying pan to cool for several minutes. When cooled, grease the frying pan with about 1 tablespoon of the olive oil. Use a spatula or large spoon to press the reserved dough evenly into the pan, tracking up the sides at least 2.5 cm (1 in). Bake for 15 minutes.

Remove the crust from the oven and top with the pizza sauce, onion and pepper mixture, pepperoni, and the remaining cheese. Drizzle with the remaining olive oil. Bake for 10 minutes, or until the cheese is melted.

Per serving: 938 calories, 32 g protein, 22 g carbohydrates, 80 g total fat, 15 g saturated fat, 9 g fiber, 1,092 mg sodium

MOZZARELLA CHEESE STICKS

For the sake of long-term family health and harmony, we are going to break one of our long-standing Wheat Belly lifestyle rules and allow a moment of deep-frying—but it's for a good cause!

The key with fried mozzarella sticks is to not let the cheese begin to liquefy from the hot oil. I've specified 30 seconds of frying time in the recipe, but be prepared to cut back just a bit. Each stick should emerge lightly browned, with its "breading" intact and the cheese a little floppy but not outright liquid.

Makes 12

Coconut oil, avocado oil, or lard

2 eggs

100 g (3½ oz) ground almonds/flour

1½ tablespoons grated Parmesan cheese

2 teaspoons dried oregano

1 teaspoon garlic powder

350 g (12 oz) block of mozzarella cheese, cut into 12 sticks

185 g (6 oz) tomato sauce (optional)

In a small frying pan wide enough to accommodate the length of the cheese sticks, pour the oil deep enough to cover the cheese. Heat to 190°C/375°F/Gas mark 5.

Meanwhile, in a medium bowl, whisk the eggs. In another medium bowl, combine the ground almonds/flour, Parmesan, oregano, and garlic powder. Mix well.

Using tongs, roll a cheese stick in the eggs, then the ground almonds/flour mixture. Fry for about 30 seconds, or until lightly browned. Transfer to a plate lined with kitchen paper to drain (this will preserve crispness). Repeat with each cheese stick.

Serve plain or with tomato sauce for dipping.

Per serving (1 stick): 154 calories, 9 g protein, 3 g carbohydrates, 12 g total fat, 5 g saturated fat, 1 g fiber, 225 mg sodium

PEANUT BUTTER COOKIES

Use the perennial favorite of kids (and husbands), peanut butter, to win them over to your grain-free side.

For an extra-special treat, dip half of each cookie into melted 85% cacao chocolate.

Makes 20

100 g (3 ½ oz) ground almonds/flour

60 g (2½ oz) finely chopped walnuts

1 teaspoon ground cinnamon

Sweetener equivalent to
170 g (6 oz) sugar

2 eggs

500 g (1 lb 2 oz) unsweetened natural
peanut butter, at room temperature

125 g (4½ oz) butter or coconut oil,
melted

1 tablespoon molasses

1 teaspoon vanilla extract

Preheat the oven to 180°C/350°F/Gas mark 4. Line a baking sheet with parchment paper.

In a large bowl, combine the ground almonds/flour, walnuts, cinnamon, and sweetener. Mix well. In a medium bowl, whisk the eggs. Add the peanut butter, butter or coconut oil, molasses, and vanilla and stir thoroughly.

Pour the peanut butter mixture into the ground almonds/flour mixture and mix thoroughly.

Spoon the dough onto the baking sheet in approximately twenty 4–5 cm (1½ in to 2 in), 2 cm (¾ in) high mounds, pressing and shaping with a large spoon. Bake for 15 minutes, or until very lightly browned.

Per serving (1 cookie): 264 calories, 8 g protein, 8 g carbohydrates, 23 g total fat, 5 g saturated fat, 2 g fiber, 146 mg sodium

KEY LIME TRUFFLES

These bite-size morsels burst with the flavor of limes. Serve them after dinner or leave them out for a snack, and they will bring any Wheat Belly naysayers to their knees.

Makes 24

240 g (8 oz) shredded unsweetened coconut

Sweetener equivalent to 230 g (8 oz) sugar

2 egg whites

225 g (8 oz) cream cheese (preferably organic), at room temperature

½ teaspoon ground cardamom (optional)

2 tablespoons lime juice

2 teaspoons grated lime peel

Preheat the oven to 150°C/300°F/Gas mark 2. Line a baking sheet with parchment paper.

In a large bowl, combine the coconut and sweetener and toss to mix thoroughly.

In another bowl, using an electric mixer on high speed, whip the egg whites until stiff peaks form. With the mixer on low speed or by hand, gently stir in the cream cheese, cardamom (if using), and lime juice. Pour the egg white mixture into the coconut mixture and mix well.

With a 2.5 cm (1 in) cookie scoop or a large spoon, scoop the mixture onto the baking sheet in 24 mounds. Sprinkle lime zest over the top of each truffle. Bake for 20 minutes, or until the truffles just begin to brown.

Per serving (1 truffle): 142 calories, 2 g protein, 4 g carbohydrates, 13 g total fat, 10 g saturated fat, 2 g fiber, 41 mg sodium

AMARETTO TRUFFLES

If you love the almond flavor of the popular liqueur amaretto, you will love these melt-in-your-mouth Amaretto Truffles. There is no alcohol, of course, so these tasty treats are appropriate for kids as well as adults. They're heavenly with coffee or hot tea.

Makes 16

240 ml (8 fl oz) whipping cream or canned coconut milk (see note)

120 g (4 oz) shredded unsweetened coconut

60 g (2½ oz) slivered almonds

Sweetener equivalent to 55 g (2 oz) sugar

1 teaspoon almond extract

In a large bowl, whisk the cream or coconut milk until stiff peaks form. With a spoon, gently stir in the coconut, almonds, sweetener, and almond extract.

With a cookie scoop or spoon, scoop the mixture onto a plate in 16 mounds and shape as desired. Refrigerate for at least 1 hour before serving.

Note: *If using canned coconut milk, refrigerate it for several hours first, then use only the solid that separates, saving the remaining water for other uses such as making Coconut Electrolyte Replacement Water (page 152).*

Per serving (1 truffle): 150 calories, 2 g protein, 4 g carbohydrates, 14 g total fat, 10 g saturated fat, 2 g fiber, 9 mg sodium

DARK CHOCOLATE COCONUT CLUSTERS

If you're prone to chocolate attacks, here is your solution. You and your family will be pleasantly surprised that such rich candies fit into a healthy lifestyle.

Use the darkest chocolate you can to minimize sugar exposure, preferably 85, 90, or even 100% cacao. (Depending on the cacao content, you'll just have to compensate with greater reliance on your choice of sweetener.)

If you replace the liquid stevia or monk fruit sweetener with a crystalline or solid sweetener, you may have to reduce it to the consistency of icing sugar by pulsing it in your food chopper or processor before adding it to the recipe. Otherwise, you could encounter a gritty consistency from the sweetener crystals.

Makes 10

225 g (8 oz) chocolate (85% cacao or greater)

30 g (1 oz) shredded unsweetened coconut

40 g (1½ oz) whole almonds

Liquid stevia or monk fruit to taste (optional)

Lay out 10 cupcake liners.

In a small microwaveable bowl, break the chocolate into fragments. Microwave on high power in 20-second increments, stirring after each interval. Alternatively, you can use a double boiler.

Stir in the coconut and almonds. Add sweetener to taste, if using. Evenly divide among the cupcake liners.

Cool in the refrigerator for at least 30 minutes before serving.

Per serving (1 cluster): 188 calories, 3 g protein, 12 g carbohydrates, 14 g total fat, 8 g saturated fat, 3 g fiber, 6 mg sodium

STRAWBERRIES 'N' CREAM MINI CHEESECAKES

All doubts over how delicious a wheat-free lifestyle can be will crumble with these irresistible mini cheesecakes served for dessert or a snack. They are also great packed into a lunch.

Makes 12

CASE

200 g (7 oz) ground almonds/flour

Sweetener equivalent to 1 tablespoon sugar

1 teaspoon ground cinnamon

60 ml (2 fl oz) coconut oil or butter, melted

FILLING

350 g (12 oz) cream cheese (preferably organic), at room temperature

225 g (8 oz) sour cream, Greek yogurt, or canned coconut milk

3 eggs

Sweetener equivalent to 170 g (6 oz) sugar

400 g (14 oz) strawberries, chopped or reduced to a pulp in a food chopper or processor

30 g (1 oz) shredded unsweetened coconut

Preheat the oven to 180°C/350°F/Gas mark 4. Place paper liners in a 12-cup muffin tin.

To make the case: In a large bowl, combine the ground almonds/flour, sweetener, cinnamon, and coconut oil or butter. Mix thoroughly. Evenly divide among the paper liners. Press flat with a spoon or your fingers. If the mixture is too crumbly or sticky to work with, chill it in the refrigerator for 20 to 30 minutes first, then press firmly with a spoon. Set aside.

To make the filling: In a large bowl, combine the cream cheese; sour cream, yogurt, or coconut milk; eggs; sweetener; and strawberries. Using an electric mixer, blend thoroughly. Evenly divide among the crusts. Bake for 25 minutes, or until lightly browned.

Sprinkle the top of each cheesecake with some of the coconut.

Per serving (1 cheesecake): 338 calories, 8 g protein, 10 g carbohydrates, 31 g total fat, 15 g saturated fat, 3 g fiber, 132 mg sodium

1-MINUTE BLUEBERRY ICE CREAM

I recognize that our effort to get away from processed food products and return to real, single-ingredient foods involves time and effort. Here is a way to make your own ice cream that requires almost no effort. Note that, for this time-saving shortcut to work, the blueberries must be frozen. And, as always, adjust the quantity of sweetener to the tastes of your family, depending on how far along the wheat-free process they have progressed.

Add a green, unripe banana to the mix if you want to add about 27 grams of prebiotic fibers to the treat.

Makes 4 servings (2 cups)

240 ml (8 fl oz) double or whipping cream or canned coconut milk

155 g (5½ oz) frozen blueberries

Sweetener equivalent to 1 tablespoon sugar

½ teaspoon vanilla extract

In a blender, combine the whipping cream or coconut milk, blueberries, sweetener, and vanilla. Blend until the mixture thickens.

Per serving (½ cup): 229 calories, 1 g protein, 7 g carbohydrates, 22 g total fat, 14 g saturated fat, 1 g fiber, 23 mg sodium

HOMEMADE IRISH CREAM

How about surprising your spouse with an after-dinner Irish Cream digestif served as is or in coffee? Here is how you re-create the popular liqueur without sugar or dairy products. If you'd like, sprinkle the top with shaved dark chocolate just before serving.

Makes 8 servings (2 cups)

3 eggs (see note)

1 can (400 g/14 oz) coconut milk

3½ tablespoons unsweetened cocoa powder

Sweetener equivalent to 115 g (4 oz) sugar

1 tablespoon instant coffee granules

½ teaspoon ground cinnamon

240 ml (8 fl oz) unflavored rum

In a blender, combine the eggs, coconut milk, cocoa, sweetener, coffee granules, cinnamon, and rum. Blend until well combined.

Store any leftovers in an airtight container in the refrigerator.

Note: *If you're concerned about the safety of raw eggs, consider using pasteurized eggs.*

Per serving (¼ cup): 202 calories, 4 g protein, 4 g carbohydrates, 13 g total fat, 10 g saturated fat, 1 g fiber, 34 mg sodium

WHEAT BELLY DETOX
WINNING LUNCHES

Lunches provide a special challenge, since most of us have become accustomed to bringing something portable to the workplace or classroom that can be delivered to the mouth with a food delivery "device," such as sandwich bread or a pita. While one solution can be to get away from such notions, carrying soup in a thermos, for instance, we can also re-create portable yet healthy alternatives that will please the kids and spouse if they carry their lunches. It can be especially helpful to have some divided plastic lunch containers or bento box sets to fill with a variety of foods.

I didn't specifically address this issue in previous *Wheat Belly* books, and readers have told me that they did a fair amount of searching for alternatives to conventional lunches. I therefore provide some easy, healthy lunch solutions here. As with all other recipes in your Secret Weapon arsenal, all the lunches provided here are consistent with the Wheat Belly detox, as well as a long-term Wheat Belly lifestyle, and can therefore be used to replace any of the lunches (or other meals, though not your Detox Shakes) in the Menu Plan. You can therefore use any of these recipes to create your own portable lunches during your detox experience, and you can also use them to pack lunches for the family.

Any sandwich can, of course, be re-created using the Wheat Belly Herbed Focaccia Bread (see page 113). That alone opens up a world of possibilities, such as Reuben sandwiches, BLT sandwiches, ham and Swiss cheese sandwiches, and egg salad sandwiches. To save on time and effort, you can make a double batch of Focaccia Bread on the weekend; if you store it in the refrigerator, it will last for several days. Some of the recipes provided in your 10-Day Menu Plan can be used as packed lunches, such as the "Potato" Salad, Apricot Ginger "Granola," Cream of Broccoli Soup, leftover Italian Sausage and Pepper Pizza, Mediterranean "Pasta" Salad, and Roasted Brussels Sprouts and Ham Fry-Up. The Detox Snack Balls are also perfect to pack for lunch. Always consider any breakfast or dinner leftovers as a lunch possibility, also.

Here are a number of other possibilities for quick, easy-to-prepare, and tasty alternatives for lunch that will help keep your kids and spouse—as well as you—on track.

TURKEY-WRAPPED PICKLES AND OLIVES. Slice a pickle in half lengthwise, wrap it in a slice of turkey meat, place an olive on top, and fix the entire stack with a wooden pick. Pack several for each lunch.

HARD-BOILED EGGS OR DEVILED EGGS. Hard-boiled or deviled eggs are perfect to pack for lunch. Also consider other egg-based dishes for lunch. For example, whenever you prepare a frittata, save the leftovers for lunches.

CHEESE. Cheeses, cut up into squares, are perfect finger foods to pack. Always look for organic *full*-fat, not skim, reduced, or low-fat.

SLICED FRUIT AND RAW VEGGIES. Kids have more leeway in their tolerance to the sugars from fruit, so sliced apples, pears, peaches, orange wedges, and other fruit easily fit into their diets. (If packing your own lunch, however, stick with berries. If you pack other fruits, such as an apple or peach, don't forget to adhere to our 15 gram net carb cutoff in order not to booby-trap your detox program.) Pack some into one of their lunch container compartments. Likewise, sliced celery, green peppers, carrots, cucumbers, and broccoli are among the choices for portable veggies. If you pack sliced fruit, consider adding a dab of peanut butter, almond butter, or other nut butter for dipping. For veggies, consider including some hummus, guacamole, ranch dressing, or salsa.

NUTS AND SEEDS. Nuts and seeds figure fairly prominently in the Wheat Belly lifestyle, and fortunately, they easily fit into packable lunches (provided that nuts are not prohibited at your child's school). Some raw or dry-roasted almonds, walnuts, pecans, macadamia nuts, pistachios, Brazil nuts, or hazelnuts in one of the lunch box compartments can be an easy and filling finger food.

HEALTHY BEVERAGES. You can find stainless steel water bottles decorated for kids in most department stores. (Avoid plastic bottles.) Fill them with a healthy drink such as homemade chocolate milk (sweetened with stevia drops), fruit-infused water, or almond or coconut milk.

SOME ADDITIONAL KID-FRIENDLY LUNCH RECIPES

CHICKEN NUGGETS

Pack these Chicken Nuggets plain or with some ketchup, honey mustard, or your child's favorite salad dressing (the least sugary option!) for dipping.

Makes 4 servings

450 g (1 lb) boneless, skinless chicken breasts

2 eggs

125 g (4½ oz) butter, melted

65 g (2½ oz) ground golden flaxseeds

25 g (1 oz) grated Parmesan cheese

½ teaspoon onion powder

Preheat the oven to 190°C/375°F/Gas mark 5. Line a baking sheet with parchment paper.

Cut the chicken into bite-size pieces.

In a small bowl, whisk the eggs and butter. In a shallow bowl, combine the flaxseeds, cheese, and onion powder. Mix well.

Coat each chicken piece in the egg mixture, then roll in the flaxseed mixture and transfer to the baking sheet.

Bake for 20 minutes, turning once, or until no longer pink and the juices run clear.

Per serving: 451 calories, 32 g protein, 5 g carbohydrates, 34 g total fat, 17 g saturated fat, 4 g fiber, 446 mg sodium

FRANKS 'N' BEANS

I've loosened the carbohydrate limit just a bit for the kids once again, since they tolerate carbs better than us big kids. Still, these Franks 'n' Beans will be heavier on the franks, lighter on the beans, but still tasty—certainly tastier than something out of a can or a frozen dinner.

Makes 4 servings

2 teaspoons butter or extra-virgin olive oil

1 medium onion, chopped

3 rashers bacon, chopped into 1 cm (½ in) pieces

1 can (425 g/15 oz) pinto beans with or without pork

2 tablespoons molasses

1 teaspoon yellow mustard

2 tablespoons tomato purée

450 g (1 lb) nitrate- and preservative-free frankfurters, sliced into 2.5 cm (1 in) pieces

In a large frying pan over medium-high heat, heat the butter or olive oil. Cook the onion and bacon for 3 minutes, or until the onion is translucent and the bacon is cooked through. Stir in the pinto beans, molasses, mustard, tomato purée, and frankfurters. Reduce the heat to low and simmer for about 5 minutes, stirring occasionally, or until heated through.

Per serving: 446 calories, 22 g protein, 27 g carbohydrates, 27 g total fat, 10 g saturated fat, 7 g fiber, 609 mg sodium

"MAC" 'N' CHEESE

This "Mac" 'n' Cheese will need to be reheated when served. You can pack it in a microwaveable container (provided your child is reliable enough to bring it back home) or just save it for a weekend lunch.

Makes 4 servings

1 head cauliflower, broken into florets and cut into 2.5 cm (1 in) pieces

¼ cup butter

375 g (13 oz) shredded Cheddar cheese

120 ml (4 fl oz) double cream

1 teaspoon dry mustard

Preheat the oven to 160°C/325°F/Gas mark 3.

Place a steamer basket in a large pot with 5 cm (2 in) of water. Bring to a boil over medium-high heat. Place the cauliflower in the basket, cover, and steam for 15 to 20 minutes, or until soft.

Meanwhile, in a large ovenproof frying pan over low heat, heat the butter, cheese, cream, and mustard, covered, stirring occasionally, for 10 minutes, or until the cheese is melted.

Transfer the cauliflower to the cheese mixture and mix well. Bake, uncovered, for 20 minutes, or until the top is lightly browned.

Per serving: 586 calories, 25 g protein, 9 g carbohydrates, 51 g total fat, 32 g saturated fat, 3 g fiber, 683 mg sodium

PIZZA ROLL-UPS

These little Pizza Roll-Ups are deceptively filling, even if only 1 or 2 fit into your child's lunch container. For a more pronounced tomato flavor, add more sun-dried tomatoes. Those soaked in olive oil work best (rather than dried).

Makes 4 servings

200 g (7 oz) ground almonds/flour

225 g (8 oz) shredded mozzarella cheese, divided

40 g (1½ oz) sun-dried tomatoes, finely chopped

2 eggs

60 ml (2 fl oz) extra-virgin olive oil

1 teaspoon dried oregano

1 teaspoon dried basil

50 g (2 oz) pepperoni, thinly sliced

Preheat the oven to 180°C/350°F/Gas mark 4. Line a baking sheet with parchment paper.

In a large bowl, combine the ground almonds/flour, two-thirds of the cheese, and the sun-dried tomatoes.

In a small bowl, whisk the eggs. Stir in the olive oil. Pour the egg mixture into the ground almonds/flour mixture and mix thoroughly until a thick dough forms.

Spread the dough out on the baking sheet to form an approximately 25 × 25 cm (10 × 10 in) square no more than 1 cm (½in) thick. (Dip your hands in oil or water to make spreading the dough easier.) Sprinkle the oregano and basil over the top. Arrange the pepperoni and then the remaining cheese over the top.

Carefully roll the dough, lifting the parchment paper from 1 end to start. Repair any tears by hand. Bake for 22 minutes, or until lightly browned.

Allow to cool for 5 minutes before slicing into 2.5 cm (1 in) thick slices.

Per serving: 728 calories, 30 g protein, 13 g carbohydrates, 62 g total fat, 12 g saturated fat, 7 g fiber, 557 mg sodium

TRAVEL AND ENTERTAINING

As we've discussed, you ideally conduct the 10 days of your detox while at home and not traveling, or at least limit travel to short day trips so that you maintain access to your own kitchen. However, should you need to travel during your detox, or desire some additional dishes after the detox period is over, maintaining a healthy wheat- and grain-free lifestyle is entirely doable. Here are some additional ideas for foods to take along with you while traveling, as well as dishes that can be useful for entertaining, even if those you are entertaining are not following this lifestyle.

Staying true to this lifestyle means ordering carefully at restaurants by choosing simple dishes such as a steak or baked fish rather than complex dishes with breading, sauces, and reductions. Even though most "gluten-free" ingredients are incompatible with the Wheat Belly lifestyle, be aware that a growing number of restaurants are serving (or at least trying to serve) gluten-free choices, and it can be helpful to play this gluten-free game. Be careful here, though: Avoid gluten-free breads, rolls, pizza, and sandwiches, as the quantity of gluten-free cornflour, potato flour, tapioca starch, and rice flour required to create these foods will reverse many of the benefits you've obtained with this lifestyle. But if, say, you request a salad or baked fish that is gluten-free (without croutons or breading), then you are likely safe, as any quantity of gluten-free ingredient is likely to be very small or negligible.

The Apricot Ginger "Granola" from the Menu Plan makes a perfect travel snack packed in resealable plastic bags or plastic containers. The Snack Balls and portable versions of the Fat Blasters in Chapter 6 also make easy-to-take-along snacks for traveling, as do many of the dishes provided as the Great Persuaders, such as the Strawberries 'n' Cream Mini Cheesecakes, Peanut Butter Cookies, Key Lime or Amaretto Truffles, and Dark Chocolate Coconut Clusters. Simply pack them in a resealable plastic container or carefully pack them in plastic wrap and keep them chilled in a cooler. The Jumbo Gingerbread Nut Muffins from the recipe in the Menu Plan are also great for travel, if packed carefully. The recipe can be altered by using conventional, rather than jumbo, muffin pans to make standard-size muffins that are easier to carry in, say, your purse or carry-on luggage.

You will also find that most of the Great Persuaders can double as useful dishes for entertaining. Your grain-consuming friends are unlikely to notice that your Chicago-Style Deep-Dish Pepperoni Pizza, Strawberries 'n' Cream Mini Cheese-cakes, or Amaretto Truffles are free of all problem ingredients (though they may notice that your dishes are unusually filling and, unlike eating elsewhere, do not result in weight gain). Likewise, many of the dishes provided in the 10-Day Menu Plan can easily be served as meals for entertaining, such as the Chorizo, Pepper, and Avocado Fry-Up served for brunch, or Bacon-Topped Meat Loaf with Mushrooms and Gravy or the Pork Thai Stir-Fry for dinner.

You can also convert many of your own favorite recipes to safe versions by adhering to the Wheat Belly Detox guidelines of using no wheat or other grains, with each serving providing no more than 15 grams net carbohydrates, and including no other problem ingredients such as added sugar, excessive use of sweeteners like honey, or unhealthy oils such as corn oil. Almond meal or flour, for example, can be substituted for conventional flour; a mixture of ground golden flaxseeds and grated Parme-san cheese can be used as "breading" on meats; and stevia or monk fruit can be used in place of sugar. A bit of trial and error may be involved, however, to get the proportions and cooking times right, as most recipes cannot be re-created with an ingredient-for-ingredient, grams for grams swap but instead require some adjustments. Nonetheless, very few dishes cannot be converted to healthier versions. (Also, see the *Wheat Belly Cookbook* and

Wheat Belly 30-Minute (or Less!) Cookbook for oodles of recipes that are useful for entertaining, as well as additional kid-friendly recipes, in which proportions and cooking times have already been worked out.)

In a world of unsafe, unhealthy processed foods, finding snack foods that are safe is a perennial challenge for us. Here are fun and tasty snacks that are easily portable to take with you while traveling. While plain raw or dry-roasted nuts can be carried as is, after that habit gets old, here are some new alternatives to carry with you when you are in an airport or during long car rides. These recipes can also be served anytime that you and your family want a snack that you can eat without worrying about negative health implications or going off your detox program.

Some safe snacks include:

- Cheese: Simply cut it into cubes and store them in a plastic container.
- Nut butters: These can be purchased in single-serve packets. Avoid purchasing those with added sugars or other unhealthy ingredients.
- Jerky: Look for the brands with the least sugar and no wheat or cornflour, of course.
- Dark chocolate: Preferably, choose varieties that are 85 percent cacao or greater.

If you are into dehydrating foods, dehydrated apples, peaches, bananas, and other fruit make excellent snacks. While fresh fruit is high in sugar, sliced dehydrated fruit tends to be consumed in much smaller quantities and is therefore a safe choice.

For even greater variety, here are a few recipes for portable snacks, or snacks that can be served to guests even if they do not engage in the same lifestyle as you. As with all of the other recipes provided here and elsewhere in this book, these snacks fit into your 10-day detox program, as well as afterward.

BERRY COCONUT CRUNCH MIX

This wonderfully easy snack provides a unique, tasty flavor and travels easily, while also looking exotic and delicious as a light snack for entertaining.

Look for the dehydrated berries in health food shops. You could, of course, dehydrate berries yourself and save considerably on cost.

Makes 8 servings

60 g (2½ oz) dehydrated cranberries, strawberries, blueberries, or other berries

220 g (7 oz) unsweetened coconut flakes

60 ml (2 fl oz) coconut oil, melted

Sweetener equivalent to 115 g (4 oz) sugar

Preheat the oven to 140°C/275°F/Gas mark 1.

In a food chopper or food processor, pulse the dehydrated berries until they're reduced to powder and small fragments.

In a large bowl, combine the powdered berries, coconut flakes, coconut oil, and sweetener. Mix thoroughly.

Spread the mixture in a shallow baking pan and bake for 14 to 16 minutes, stirring once, or until very lightly browned. Be careful not to allow the coconut to burn.

Per serving: 391 calories, 3 g protein, 13 g carbohydrates, 36 g total fat, 31 g saturated fat, 6 g fiber, 14 mg sodium

DARK CHOCOLATE–DIPPED COCONUT MACAROONS

Carry a few of these rich macaroons on trips to fill you and your family up. Or serve them to family and friends as a light dessert after a meal. You should hear no complaints about missing candy bars or ice cream!

Makes 8

3 egg whites

120 g (4 oz) shredded unsweetened coconut

Sweetener equivalent to 115 g (4 oz) sugar

110 g (4 oz) chocolate (85% cacao or greater), broken into pieces

Preheat the oven to 180°C/350°F/Gas mark 4. Line a baking sheet with parchment paper.

In a large bowl, using an electric mixer on high speed, beat the egg whites until stiff peaks form. Gently fold the coconut and sweetener into the egg white mixture.

Scoop the mixture onto the baking sheet to form 8 mounds. Bake for 15 minutes, or until golden and slightly firm to the touch. Allow to cool.

Meanwhile, in a small microwaveable bowl, microwave the chocolate on high power in 15-second increments, stirring after each interval, until melted. Alternatively, melt the chocolate in a double boiler. Carefully dip the bottom third of each macaroon into the chocolate and place back on the parchment paper to cool.

Per serving (1 macaroon): 254 calories, 4 g protein, 13 g carbohydrates, 21 g total fat, 16 g saturated fat, 4 g fiber, 30 mg sodium

CHOCOLATE CRACKERS

Making your own crackers involves a bit of work, certainly more than tearing open a package of Ritz crackers and dipping in. But these delicious crackers dipped in dark chocolate are well worth it.

If you're packing the crackers for traveling, keep them cool so that the chocolate doesn't melt. I've specified 85% cacao chocolate, but you can add additional liquid sweetener, such as liquid stevia or monk fruit, to sweeten it up if, say, kids will be eating them.

Makes approximately 24

200 g (7 oz) almond flour

30 g (1 oz) coconut flour

Sweetener equivalent to 115 g (4 oz) sugar

½ teaspoon sea salt

1 teaspoon ground cinnamon

1 teaspoon bicarbonate of soda

2 eggs

120 ml (4fl oz) coconut, almond, or hemp milk

2 teaspoons vanilla extract

60 g (2½ oz) butter, cold and sliced

110 g (4 oz) chocolate (85% cacao), broken into pieces

Line a baking sheet with parchment paper.

In a large bowl, combine the almond flour, coconut flour, sweetener, salt, cinnamon, and bicarbonate of soda. Mix well.

In a cup or small bowl, whisk the eggs. Add the milk and vanilla and mix well. Add the egg mixture to the almond flour mixture and mix thoroughly. Cut in the butter using a pastry blender or fork. Form into a large ball, wrap in clingfilm, and refrigerate for 30 minutes.

Preheat the oven to 180°C/350°F/Gas mark 4.

Place the unwrapped dough on the baking sheet. Flatten to about a
2.5 mm (⅛ in) thickness with a rolling pin. (If the dough sticks to the rolling
pin, use a second sheet of parchment paper on top and remove it before baking.)

Bake for 30 minutes, or until lightly browned at the edges. Cool. Using a pastry
or pizza cutter, cut into desired shapes and sizes.

In a small microwaveable bowl, microwave the chocolate on high power in
15-second increments, stirring after each interval, until melted. Alternatively,
melt it in a double boiler and then transfer the melted chocolate to a small bowl.
Carefully dip each cracker into the chocolate until half covered, then place on a
platter or large plate lined with greaseproof paper. Refrigerate for at least 10
minutes before serving.

*Per serving (1 cracker): 120 calories, 3 g protein, 5 g carbohydrates, 10 g total fat,
3 g saturated fat, 2 g fiber, 112 mg sodium*

CHIPOTLE CHILLI CRACKERS

Pack these spicy Chipotle Chilli Crackers for your next trip and bring along a small container of hummus, salsa, guacamole, or artichoke dip for dipping. Be sure to examine the label of the chipotle seasoning you choose and avoid those with any problem ingredients, such as "modified food starch."

Makes approximately 20

130 g (4½ oz) finely ground golden flaxseeds

50 g (2 oz) grated Parmesan cheese

1 teaspoon sea salt

1 tablespoon chipotle seasoning

1 teaspoon onion powder

½ teaspoon cayenne pepper

300 ml (11 fl oz) water

Preheat the oven to 190°C/375°F/Gas mark 5. Grease a 28 × 20 cm (11 × 8 in) shallow baking pan.

In a large bowl, combine the flaxseeds, cheese, salt, chipotle seasoning, onion powder, and cayenne pepper. Mix well.

Pour in the water and mix *quickly* until just combined. Pour into the baking pan and spread evenly. If the dough begins to firm up before you can spread it, use a large spoon, wetted under hot water if necessary, to spread the dough to a uniform thickness.

Bake for 15 minutes. Turn the oven off but leave the pan in the oven for an additional 30 minutes. Remove from oven and, using a pizza cutter, cut into about 20 crackers.

Per serving (1 cracker): 34 calories, 2 g protein, 2 g carbohydrates, 2 g total fat, 0.5 g saturated fat, 2 g fiber, 167 mg sodium

HOT AND SPICY NUT MIX

Have a glass of water nearby when you eat these nuts. Pack this Hot and Spicy Nut Mix in a resealable plastic bag or plastic container and take it along with you when you travel. It's certainly tastier and a lot less expensive than the nuts sold at airports or other travel shops. If making it for the kids, add cashew fragments to your choice of nuts. (Adult versions should avoid cashews or minimize them due to potentially excessive carbohydrate exposure.)

If you start with whole nuts, you can reduce them to smaller pieces in your food chopper, food processor, or coffee grinder by pulsing briefly.

Makes 16 servings

130 g (4½ oz) raw pumpkin seeds

125 g (4½ oz) raw sunflower seeds

125 g (4½ oz) raw walnut pieces

125 g (4½ oz) raw pecan pieces

120 ml (4 fl oz) cup coconut oil, melted

1 tablespoon chilli powder

2 tablespoons hot-pepper sauce

½ teaspoon sea salt

Preheat the oven to 140°C/275°F/Gas mark 1.

In a large bowl, combine the pumpkin seeds, sunflower seeds, walnuts, pecans, coconut oil, chilli powder, hot sauce, and salt. Toss to mix thoroughly.

Spread the mixture on a large baking sheet. Bake for 20 minutes, stirring once. Cool before serving.

Per serving: 253 calories, 6 g protein, 5 g carbohydrates, 24 g total fat, 8 g saturated fat, 2 g fiber, 97 mg sodium

"HONEY" NUT MIX

Here's a slightly sweet nut mix to pack for travel or use as a breakfast cereal. Despite the name, there's no real honey in this recipe, only the taste and feel of it. If you're making it for the kids, add cashew fragments to your choice of nuts. (Adult versions should avoid cashews or minimize them due to potentially excessive carbohydrate exposure.)

If you start with whole nuts, you can reduce them to smaller pieces in your food chopper, food processor, or coffee grinder by pulsing briefly.

Makes 24 servings (6 cups)

1 cup raw pumpkin seeds

125 g (4½ oz) raw sunflower seeds

125 g (4½ oz) raw walnut pieces

125 g (4½ oz) raw pecan pieces

120 ml (4 fl oz) coconut oil, melted

120 g (4 oz) shredded unsweetened coconut

1 teaspoon vanilla extract

2 teaspoons ground cinnamon

1 teaspoon ground nutmeg

½ teaspoon ground cloves

Sweetener equivalent to 2 teaspoons sugar

Preheat the oven to 140°C/275°F/Gas mark 1.

In a large bowl, combine the pumpkin seeds, sunflower seeds, walnuts, pecans, coconut oil, shredded coconut, vanilla, cinnamon, nutmeg, cloves, and sweetener. Toss to mix thoroughly.

Spread the mixture on a large baking sheet. Bake for 20 minutes, stirring once. Cool before serving.

Per serving: 232 calories, 5 g protein, 5 g carbohydrates, 23 g total fat, 10 g saturated fat, 2 g fiber, 4 mg sodium

STILL NOT CONVERTED?

What if you've launched the Wheat Belly Detox Secret Weapons to convert the unconverted, yet they remain stubbornly unconvinced that this lifestyle is the most powerful thing that has come along to reachieve health and weight in, oh, the last 10,000 years?

Well, then you will need the tincture of time. There may be reasons that the people close to you remain resistant: They may be unwilling to confront their addiction to gliadin protein–containing grains and the withdrawal process that follows their elimination; they may—incredibly—still fear that they will be deprived of tasty comfort foods; or they may be reluctant to accept the fact that so much conventional nutritional advice is worthless, even destructive, dashing their faith in advice from "higher" sources.

Preparing dishes consistent with the Wheat Belly lifestyle will usually go unnoticed by most family members. In other words, if you prepared, say, chicken wings or a stir-fry that adheres to the Wheat Belly principles, most family members will simply enjoy the meal and *never even notice*. They may not agree with the dietary approach you are following, but they can certainly enjoy the wonderful foods you prepare.

Secret weapons or no, the most important persuader remains observing *your* success. If they observe you losing, say, 43 pounds without trying, taking on an entirely new physical appearance because you have divorced yourself from the inflammation, water retention, and added pounds of grain consumption, while regaining energy and vigor that you thought you'd lost 20 years earlier, well, how can they *not* notice? They may also observe that you are eating rich, delicious foods without worrying about calories or portion size and not gaining a pound, while they seem to struggle with weight gain, fatigue, and dependence on prescription drugs. Witnessing your transformation and that of anyone else around you who embraces this lifestyle should, over time, open their eyes. *You* are therefore the ultimate secret weapon of persuasion to adopt this empowering lifestyle.

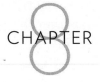

CHAPTER 8

BEYOND THE GRAINS: ADDITIONAL IMPORTANT HEALTH SITUATIONS YOU SHOULD KNOW ABOUT

THERE ARE A number of important changes in your body that will get under way during your Wheat Belly 10-Day Detox—some profound, some subtle, but all good, all reflecting the physiologic changes that develop after removing wheat and grains and correcting residual health effects left in their wake. Like tainted well water that poisons an entire village, removing the poison promptly allows everyone to start recovering.

But here's the challenge: Unlike the obvious relief that results from avoiding tainted water, your body may change in such unique and unexpected ways that you may not even recognize them as being the result of the detox process. The damaging health effects of wheat and grains are so wide and far reaching— from the foot pain of plantar fasciitis and the repeated accumulation of dental plaque to swallowed food getting painfully stuck on its way to the stomach—that most people don't even realize that these are among the consequences of wheat and grain consumption that disappear with their removal.

So let's discuss many of the body changes that you may experience that result from banishing the bran cereal, bagels, popcorn, and tacos from your life. If you better understand the benefits you obtain with this lifestyle, you will better appreciate how far off your health and appearance were diverted by wheat and grains, and be more motivated than ever to never wander back down that path. Life goes on after the detox process as you continue the detox principles in your long-term Wheat Belly lifestyle, and it helps to understand that health gets better and better in so many wonderful ways the longer you follow this lifesyle. There are also some additional issues to discuss, such as what to do with prescription medications, the peculiar issue of grain reexposure, and how to manage weight-loss plateaus.

ALEXANDRIA, 42, homemaker, Connecticut

Alexandria reported experiencing many headaches, irritability, and low energy for the first 3 days of her detox. She managed to deal with the headaches with a combination of ibuprofen, hydration, and broths for the salt.

By Day 4, she reported that mental "fuzziness" was gone, the previous difficulty she'd had with swallowing disappeared, and she was relieved of bloating after eating. "One of the biggest positive effects," she says, "was the stopping of impulsive, unstoppable, out-of-control eating. This was huge."

By the end of her detox experience, Alexandria had lost 7.3 pounds and gained a substantial improvement in mood.

MIRROR, MIRROR . . .

As you proceed through your Wheat Belly 10-Day Detox, you are likely to see some changes when you look in the mirror, changes you'll find empowering, encouraging, even thrilling. While weight loss, of course, brings its own collection of improvements, there is more that changes in some wonderful ways.

Yes, if you lose, say, 5 to 7 pounds over the 10 days of your detox, your face is going to look thinner. But you will likely notice that your face changed more than those few pounds would explain. You may observe reduced swelling or edema over your entire face and reduced puffiness around your eyes. If you compare your before-and-after photos, you may notice that your eyes look larger. If you started with redness or the wheat/grain signature seborrheic rash on your cheeks or along the sides of your nose, you will likely see this rash recede, then disappear, during the first week. Facial contours will change more than you expect, with sharpening of the jawline and cheekbones. Don't be surprised if friends ask whether you've undergone expert cosmetic surgery to achieve such dramatic effects. These are the changes that lead people on Wheat Belly social media to say that the before-and-after pictures look like two different people. (The photos are of the same person, of course, but the contrast reflects the often breathtaking transformations of this unique anti-inflammatory lifestyle.)

Be prepared to buy smaller belts as well as pants and skirts many inches smaller. Of all areas of the body that shrink in size, it's the waistline that shrinks most, reflecting the loss of inflammatory visceral fat created by grain consumption. Sometimes the deflation of abdominal size is dramatic, beginning even during the first few days, reflecting healing of the gastrointestinal tract and reduced bloating from the removal of bowel-disrupting grains, as well as loss of fat. Over days, weeks, and months, visceral fat continues its retreat, a wonderful effect that compounds the health benefits that develop in the wake of wheat and grain removal while sparing you any more questions about when you are "due."

You may also observe the following:

- **Loss of cellulite.** Many women experience a reduction or elimination of the cellulite on their thighs, a curious development that can have dramatic effects on the appearance of the legs. The retreat of cellulite can begin during the 10 days of your detox and continue over a longer period.

- **Thicker hair.** People experience thicker hair over time. Because hair grows slowly, this effect will take longer than the 10 days of your detox to notice. Women with thin patches typically experience a gradual filling in. (Men generally do not enjoy this effect, unfortunately, since male hair loss develops for different reasons.) Much less commonly, some people experience hair loss early in the process, but then their hair grows back thicker and fuller over time. This likely reflects the reversal of skin inflammation with wheat and grain removal followed by a regrowth phenomenon.

- **Changes in your nails.** Fingernails and toenails often become thicker and smoother over time as they grow, reflecting the improvement in skin health along with hair (since nails and hair are really forms of skin). Many report that fungal toenail infections—evidenced by chronic discoloration, thickening, and nail separation and usually treated with toxic medication—recede and disappear.

- **Teeth improvements.** I predict that you will experience dramatic changes in dental health: improvement in gum health and gingivitis and less plaque formation. Incredibly, even breath can change for the better, a reflection of the change in oral flora that parallels the shift in bowel flora (see pages 197–199).

- **Breast changes.** Breast size can be reduced a cup size or two, changes that are not explained by weight loss alone. While the effect is variable, this phenomenon is due to correction of hormonal distortions, especially reductions of the formerly high levels of estrogen and prolactin (prolactin = pro + lactation, meaning a hormone that encourages breast growth) with removal of grains. While some women may find this undesirable, recognize that the abnormal stimulation of breast tissue from grain consumption, compounded by the hormonal distortions of visceral fat, are risk factors for breast cancer, now corrected with grain elimination. Males, of course, celebrate the reversal of this embarrassing situation.

This is why I describe the detoxification process from wheat and grains as a head-to-toe total body makeover, as there is no organ system or body part that does not change for the better in some way, from hair to toenails. Add it all up and you have the formula for a dramatic change in appearance.

Here's a happy dilemma: How do you manage your wardrobe if you have this wonderful problem of needing smaller and smaller dress, pants, jeans, and shirt sizes? If you lose 5 pounds during your 10-day detox initiation, then another 12 pounds the rest of that month, then 20 pounds over the next several months, and 55 pounds over a year, how do you accommodate such evolving changes? Most people, of course, still have clothes from their thinner days in the back of the closet. It's worth pulling those out. I've seen other people put clothes, such as jeans, in the dryer to get them to shrink, or use thrift shops and discount stores to buy clothes they may need for only a matter of weeks or months to tide them over. Some choose pants or skirts with elastic waists or drawstrings, new belts that cinch in farther, and stretchable pants and tops. It may be worth having some of your nicer pieces, such as dresses, coats, or suits, tailored to fit as you approach your goal weight. It will indeed be necessary at some point to commit to new clothes to fit your new size and simply risk continuing changes. Unlike diets and weight-loss drugs that result in weight loss only to allow weight *regain* once you go off of them, living the Wheat Belly lifestyle is a sustainable way to maintain your goal weight once achieved. The new wardrobe is likely to be one that fits for a long time, even in low single-digit sizes.

Let's now describe further some of the other unique changes that may develop during your Wheat Belly 10-Day Detox.

MENSTRUAL FOLLIES

If you are having menstrual cycles, there can be changes in the timing of your cycle, as well as in their intensity and the amount of discomfort and bleeding as you engage in this lifestyle. While our 10-day timeline is obviously too short to experience the full range of changes that can develop, you may nonetheless notice a difference as soon as your next cycle.

Wheat and grains can be blamed for making cycles more painful and irregular, worsening premenstrual emotional symptoms, and even affecting fertility. By removing wheat and grains, you are removing these hormonal disrupters and the many abnormal phenomena they provoked, month after month, year after year. With wheat and grain elimination, cycles become more regular, often with reduced discomfort, anger, irritation, and other emotional excesses; over time, even fertility can be restored. The benefits of this lifestyle are compounded further as visceral fat is lost, recognized as a shrinking waistline and reduced body-wide inflammation (such as that reflected on the face), removing the hormonal distortions introduced by inflammatory fat.

Women with polycystic ovarian syndrome (PCOS) will notice the same sorts of changes, though to a greater degree, especially as visceral fat dissolves. Anyone with PCOS will need to keep their health care provider in the loop, as there will be a need to rapidly reduce any blood pressure or diabetes medications being taken to avoid low blood pressure or low blood sugar as your body changes. (See "How to Manage Prescription Medications" on page 200.) I have witnessed many women with PCOS completely turn off all the abnormal health phenomena of the condition with the strategies discussed in the Wheat Belly 10-Day Detox program, including the so-called masculinizing features of excess body hair, benefits that develop from receding insulin and inflammation.

Women in the perimenopausal or menopausal phases of life often report reduction in the intensity of hot flashes, occasionally experiencing complete relief. Most report improved mood, and many report increased sexual interest. While women have lower levels of testosterone than males, women can experience a rise in testosterone levels (just like the guys) and a reduction in estrogen, phenomena that account for improved mood, assertiveness, and sexual desire.

Hormonal corrections play out over a period longer than the 10 days of your detox. But recognize these changes as a shift back to the way it was supposed to be all along.

LET'S NOT FORGET THE GUYS

Let's face it: Guys are less likely to engage in discussions about health, certainly anything beyond exercise. But they stand to gain as much as women do by following the strategies discussed here. Guys have this strange affliction called "I've gotta die of something" that causes them to pooh-pooh the value of any health habit. Well, it's rarely as clean and easy as that. Life for an aging male is much more commonly that of progressive weight gain; acquiring a collection of prescription medications for blood pressure, high cholesterol, failing libido, and erectile dysfunction; and years of becoming more and more dependent on the medical system, medical procedures, and, eventually, their wives.

Because of the peculiar male attitude toward health, the majority of people engaged in the Wheat Belly 10-Day Detox process are women, and I therefore focus most of my comments on the female perspective. But I also recognize that many women are interested in learning more for the benefit of their male partners. And then there may be the occasional brave and fearless guy who is actually reading this book.

Just as women undergo tidal waves of hormonal changes as they proceed through this lifestyle, so can males. Male breasts, as mentioned above—a common sight in combination with visceral fat and surely an embarrassing feature that many men work hard to conceal—recede in parallel with a shrinking belly and waistline. Visceral fat contains high levels of an enzyme called aromatase that converts testosterone to estrogen, thereby resulting in low testosterone levels and high estrogen. Parallel to the situation in women, the A5 pentapeptide opiate that results from digestion of the gliadin protein of wheat has the unique ability to stimulate prolactin release from the pituitary gland, the hormone of pregnancy and lactation—but in males, a reflection of just how perversely grains affect us and are hormonally disruptive.

Remove wheat and grains and visceral fat recedes, aromatase activity drops, the A5 pentapeptide is no longer available to stimulate breast growth, and wonderful things happen: Man breasts shrink, testosterone goes up, estrogen goes down, libido returns, and capacity for erections can be restored. Throw in the improved vascular (blood vessel) health that results from this lifestyle, and you have the dietary equivalent of an erection-enhancing drug. (Vitamin D restoration and omega-3 fatty acids from fish oil are also important components of this equation, both of which contribute to vascular health. Both nutrients are discussed in Chapter 4.)

Men therefore experience just as many benefits as women, though somewhat different because of differing hormonal circumstances. For a man to know that a shrinking tummy and breasts, along with enhanced capacity for erections, are among the changes that develop with this lifestyle can be highly motivating. We'll just keep the big "I told you so" to ourselves.

KELLY, 47, registered nurse, Massachusetts

"Between Days 5 and 7, I noticed an increased level of energy and mood. I noticed my joints (knees and hips) were no longer bothering me. I also saw my mental clarity and focus increase at work and home. Sleep has been amazing, and I want to work out! At work, my mood and energy level were noticed as well as my skin and thinner, less puffy face."

By Day 10 of her detox experience, Kelly had lost 8.1 pounds, 3.8 percent of her starting body weight.

THE SCOOP ON POOP

Some important changes are going to occur in the region of your body just below your diaphragm as you proceed through the detox experience. While the healing of your poor grain-battered gastrointestinal tract largely occurs on its own with wheat and grain elimination, there are issues to address specifically that ensure and accelerate your healing process.

During your wheat- and grain-consuming days, your gastrointestinal tract was a battleground, enduring a continual onslaught of toxic effects. Now it can begin its healing process to undo common conditions such as esophagitis, acid reflux, gastritis, vitamin B_{12} deficiency (from damage to stomach cells that assist in B_{12} absorption), chronic constipation, and irritable bowel syndrome. For many people, relief from, say, acid reflux or bowel urgency can be rapid, occurring within the first 5 days of the detox. For others, however, healing develops over weeks to months.

A crucial part of the healing process is to restore normal bowel flora. We now appreciate just how critical the composition of bowel flora can be, despite years of dismissing it as nothing more than a curiosity. Grains are disruptive to bowel flora; now that they are removed, you will need to replace the unhealthy bowel flora with healthy species. This is why, in Chapter 4, we discussed how to "seed" your intestinal tract with healthy bacterial species from high-potency probiotic supplements, then how to nourish and cultivate these species using prebiotic fibers or resistant starches, easily obtained with the Detox Shake recipes found in Chapter 5.

Before we understood that disrupted bowel flora needed to be corrected, it was common to experience constipation during the first few weeks of giving up wheat and grains. The high-potency probiotic of the detox is your up-front remedy, repopulating the intestines with species that assist in creating regular bowel movements, while prebiotic fibers—not cellulose, as is often advised by conventional-thinking doctors and dietitians—provide a healthy solution to maintaining regular, effortless bowel movements as well as a long list of other health benefits. Following this formula, even people who were plagued by chronic struggles with constipation rediscover comfortable regularity.

An occasional person does not do well with the probiotic/prebiotic formula, experiencing bloating, diarrhea, or discomfort even after adhering to the program for several weeks. This is usually due to bowel flora that was so severely disrupted prior to initiating the detox that it resists correction and cannot be undone by these simple, natural efforts (this condition is called dysbiosis or small intestinal bacterial overgrowth, signifying that unhealthy bacteria and other organisms have climbed up the small intestine where they do not belong). In such exceptional cases, a stool analysis and other analyses should be seriously considered (meaning you will need a functional medicine practitioner or naturopath, not a gastroenterologist who just wants to scope everything in sight). The problem is often remedied with a course of antibiotics or antifungal treatments to clear the intestines of the unwanted overgrowth and start with a clean "slate." While this condition is uncommon, it is important to recognize and address it in order to resume your path back to health.

Many people struggle to give up the notion of having to supplement fibers every day to "bulk up" their bowel movements. But recall that bulking up stools with cellulose—wood fiber—is not how humans did it while living in the wild and following traditional lifestyles free of gastrointestinal struggles. Human bowel health was not maintained by consuming fiber-rich breakfast cereal or taking daily fiber supplements, but by consuming fiber from vegetables, fruits, nuts, and seeds, as well as the crucially important prebiotic fibers from legumes and underground tubers. It's the prebiotic fibers that underlie true bowel health, not cellulose. Bulkier stools can be obtained through sources such as psyllium seed or ground flaxseeds, but they are not necessary for the majority of people following this lifestyle who have taken the effort to cultivate healthy bowel flora using the strategies discussed here. I'll say it over and over again: Take care of bowel flora, and it will take care of you. If only human relationships could be as manageable.

Rarely are special allowances necessary to accommodate this lifestyle. Even if you've had years of irritable bowel struggles and had to run to the toilet to avoid accidents, or have had your gallbladder removed, following these strategies restores normal bowel function and habits in the majority. If you are among the exceptions and continue to struggle with bowel symptoms despite these efforts, then a formal evaluation by your health care provider (to identify conditions such as poor stomach acid, called hypochlorhydria, or lack of pancreatic enzymes, situations discussed in *Wheat Belly Total Health*) is in order before you can be put back on track to full bowel health.

THAT'S A MOUTHFUL

Did you know that dental problems such as cavities, gingivitis, abscesses, tooth loss, and misaligned teeth were uncommon before humans first began to consume grains? This simple fact has been understood by anthropologists studying primitive humans for decades, an observation all the more astounding when you consider that primitive people had no toothbrushes, fluoridated water, toothpaste, dental floss, or dentists—and were armed with no tools for dental hygiene other than a twig—yet reached old age with straight, intact mouths of teeth (a crucial observation on dental health, by the way, that has been ignored by most modern dentists).

Interestingly, you will re-create this experience in effortless dental health. By removing wheat and grains, you will notice—

and so will your dental hygienist and dentist—that far less plaque will need to be cleaned from your teeth, breath will improve, gingivitis will recede, and cavities will become much less common. Healthy changes in oral flora, just as with bowel flora, will develop over time, contributing to reduction in dental decay. Changes in oral flora help maintain dental health, as well as provide benefits outside the mouth (e.g., helping to maintain normal blood pressure, since by-products of bacterial metabolism influence blood pressure).

I would not suggest that you mimic the oral hygiene habits of primitive people, picking the fragments of wild boar from between your teeth with a stick and not brushing or flossing. But it means that your new lifestyle, compounded by daily oral hygiene efforts, is likely to yield a level of dental health that makes the need for dental procedures a rarity. (Here's an interesting speculation: If children are raised grain-free, will they grow up with straight, perfectly aligned teeth, without the need to have cavities filled or wear braces? It's an untested proposition, but it would mimic what is witnessed in non-grain-consuming primitive cultures whose people survive to old age with full mouths of straight, undecayed teeth, having spent not a penny on the newest toothpaste or dental insurance.)

HOW TO MANAGE PRESCRIPTION MEDICATIONS

Many people begin their Wheat Belly 10-Day Detox experience while taking medications for high blood pressure, high blood sugar, acid reflux, irritable bowel syndrome, joint pain, painful menstrual cycles, high cholesterol, depression, anxiety, or other conditions, many of which are going to recede with this lifestyle change. This means that the drugs may no longer be necessary, exposing you to only side effects without benefit. It is very common to be taking multiple prescription medications, all inadvertently prescribed to treat the consequences of what was nothing more than wheat and grain consumption. Remove the wheat and grains, and the need for many, if not most, medications evaporates. It is not uncommon to start this process with five, six, or seven prescriptions that, over time, are reduced to none. This alone makes pharmaceutical company executives sweat and reach for their Tums.

But how do you manage this with a health care provider who prescribed the medications in the first place while telling you that a diet full of "healthy whole grains" was the ticket to health? While for some the answer can be a new doctor, it is still worth going back to the initial prescriber to show them what you have accomplished.

If, for instance, you are on two blood pressure medications that have kept your blood pressure around 140/90, but minus grains it's now 102/70, it is most definitely time to start removing the medications. Most doctors will understand this and go along with stopping, say, the hydrochlorothiazide diuretic or other agent, even if they may not understand why your new lifestyle has accomplished this change. From a blood pressure viewpoint, serious consideration to reducing or stopping medications should be given if blood pressure is at or below 100/80, as we want to absolutely avoid low blood pressure that can result in effects such as light-headedness or passing out. It is important to work with your doctor or other health care provider, as some medications— especially beta-blockers such as atenolol, metoprolol, and carvedilol, and others such as clonidine—need to be withdrawn gradually and not stopped abruptly.

Another potential hazard is encountered with some medications for diabetes, especially injectable insulin and oral drugs glyburide, glipizide, and glimepiride, or when several diabetes drugs are used in combination. (Not all diabetes medications cause hypoglycemia when taken as a single agent.) When you eliminate wheat and grains, you are eliminating major contributors to high blood sugar, making the drugs less necessary to keep blood sugar down. You absolutely need to avoid hypoglycemia, or low blood sugar, since blood sugars of 4 mmol/L or less can be dangerous (resulting in losing consciousness, for instance). For this reason, if blood sugars approach 5 mmol/L or lower, it is time to have a serious discussion with your doctor as soon as possible about reducing or removing diabetes medications, especially those mentioned above that can cause hypoglycemia. Once again, your doctor may not understand how or why your blood sugars are plummeting, since you've defied his or her advice to cut fat and eat more "healthy whole grains," but you will need to politely insist on considering a reduction in medications. If you encounter skepticism, antagonism, or criticism, find a doctor who understands that becoming less diabetic or nondiabetic is a *good* thing, a major health accomplishment, and that you deserve every bit as much attention as someone obtaining the diagnosis in the first place.

Other situations, such as drugs for acid reflux, joint pain, or high cholesterol, all need to be pursued individually but are not as urgent as the issues surrounding drugs for blood pressure or diabetes. But the same principle applies: Work with a doctor who is willing and able to recognize that you are getting healthier and that the "need" for drugs is withdrawing like a receding tidal wave. You should have absolutely no qualms over finding a new doctor if the old one proves disinterested, ignorant, or critical of your newfound health.

Another happy situation can develop as you trim away some drugs, especially beta-blockers such as metoprolol or atenolol, insulin, antidepressants, and antihistamines for allergy: Weight loss proceeds even faster, since all of these common drugs either block weight loss or cause weight gain (see "Prescription Drugs That Ambush Weight Loss" on page 209).

GOING OFF COURSE

It is important that during the Wheat Belly 10-Day Detox experience, you do not wander off the program to have a few bites of your daughter's birthday cake or a slice of pizza served at work. This is because a minor "indulgence" will cause all of the unhealthy and uncontrollable phenomena of wheat and grains to be reignited. That harmless-looking cake or pizza will set you back and force you to start all over again. The appetite-stimulating effect alone can last for several days, making it tough to control food choices, and even cause weight regain, typically causing several pounds to come right back, out of proportion to the few calories you may have taken in from the exposure (since water retention and inflammation are part of the regain process). Many people even have to go through the withdrawal process again and endure several days of unpleasant feelings. There is simply no indulgence that is worth the sacrifice. It is no different than an alcoholic who persuades herself that just one or two drinks can't hurt—they do, and all benefits are lost. And get rid of crippling notions such as "everything in moderation" or "a little bit can't hurt."

The most common grain reexposure experience involves bloating, diarrhea, abdominal discomfort, joint pain, depression, headache, and the recurrence of any symptoms you previously experienced due to wheat and grains before giving them up. This can be particularly awful if you have an autoimmune or neurological condition, such as rheumatoid arthritis or peripheral neuropathy. While these conditions recede over months, they can recur and last for weeks to months with reexposure to wheat and grains. Once again, it's simply not worth it. (I've witnessed people with rheumatoid arthritis, for instance, reignite the pain and swelling of this condition with a single slice of bread, then require 6 months of grain-free living to obtain relief.)

It is especially not worth it because you can re-create nearly all wheat- and grain-based dishes with healthy recipes, such as those contained in this book. You do not have to give up pizza or cheesecake, for instance, but you can enjoy healthy versions simply by drawing from a different list of ingredients. Have the pizza or cheesecake from these recipes and there will be no headache, no diarrhea, no re-provocation of appetite, and no recurrence of prior symptoms. You can just have your grain-free pizza or cheesecake and not pay any health price.

If you have a reexposure, accidental or intentional, then you will have to go back to square one and restart your Wheat Belly 10-Day Detox.

WHAT IF THE SCALE DOESN'T BUDGE?

What should you do if you survived the emotional and physical agony of withdrawal, managed to annoy the heck out of friends and family in the process, and obtained benefits such as reduced blood sugar and relief from joint pain and bowel urgency, but failed to see the pounds drop off? It is not the most common experience, but it does happen. And it happens often enough that it is worth addressing.

First of all, make sure you are indeed following all the strategies contained here. For instance, many people discover that they are getting exposed to wheat and grains in some condiment, snack, or other food that continues to stimulate appetite and inflammation, even foods you thought would never contain grains, such as a seasoning mix, broth, or tomato sauce. Also take a look at your nutritional supplements, protein or energy drinks, and prescription drugs to identify hidden wheat and grain sources that have the potential to stimulate appetite. Even a tiny exposure can be sufficient to impair your entire detox process. Consult labels on nutritional supplements and see Appendix B for some resources to help answer questions about prescription drugs.

If you've continued old habits, such as eating a whole piece of fruit twice a day, then you have been exposing yourself to carbohydrates and sugars sufficient to trigger insulin and turn off any hope of weight loss. Yes, an apple a day turns off the ability to lose weight. Refer back to Chapter 2 to refresh your memory on carbohydrate counting and make the correction. (Eat no more than half an apple, for instance, to stay below our 15 g net carbohydrate per meal cutoff.)

If you have indeed carefully followed the advice we've included, but aren't seeing the scale drop, then consider the issues in the checklist below. The strategies in this detox are extremely powerful, but they cannot undo, for instance, the weight-loss-blocking effects of some prescription drugs or low thyroid hormone activity created by iodine deficiency. The issues in this checklist can also be helpful if you lose, say, an initial 20 pounds, only to hit a plateau that lasts for several weeks or longer. Removing the barrier can allow healthy weight loss to proceed.

When encountering resistance to weight loss, consider:

Embrace the Fat

Giving up your fear of fats and oils can be tough, given the brainwashing we've all suffered from the repeated advice to "cut your fat and cholesterol," "cut saturated fat," "avoid artery-clogging fats," etc. You have to give it up because none of this is true. Adhering to these fictions impairs weight loss, not to mention makes reversing health conditions, such as diabetes and fatty liver, tougher or impossible. The misinterpretations, bad science, and profiteering that drove the hugely destructive low-fat era is detailed in *Wheat Belly Total Health*. Rest assured that the "science" purported to support the idea of reducing fat intake was nearly nonexistent in the first place. It is among the biggest blunders in the history of dietary advice, along with the "healthy whole grain" message.

Fat does not make you fat; fat helps make you thin, and failing to embrace this concept can impair your ability to gain control over appetite and weight. This message is entirely lost, for instance, on many popular TV chefs in which the well-meaning host turns a high-fat, high-calorie dish into a low-fat or nonfat and lower-calorie one, proudly proclaiming that this remade version will help you lose weight and be healthier. It's absolute, utter nonsense. (Of course, the chef making such claims typically sports a substantial wheat belly, the signature of a fat-deprived, grain-heavy lifestyle.)

You should have already cleared your shelves of all low-fat and nonfat foods. When you buy meats, don't be afraid of buying fatty cuts, including less expensive ground meats with greater fat content. Don't trim the fat off the meats—eat it. Bacon and sausage? Go right ahead. Use healthy oils like coconut, olive oil, organic butter, and avocado oil, and use them liberally. Don't toss out the oils remaining after cooking meats; save them for reuse (in the refrigerator). Buy lard and tallow, if you can find nonhydrogenated versions. And don't be afraid to pack a bit of healthy oil for travel or eating outside the home (e.g., a small bottle of olive oil, a small container of coconut oil, or even a Fat Blaster or two).

Fats and oils induce satiety (a sense of fullness) without triggering insulin. Even high intakes of protein can provoke insulin (though not as vigorously as grains or other carbohydrates). But fat does not. Fat is therefore the perfect weight-loss food. This is one of the reasons why the Wheat Belly Detox Shakes have plentiful fat, around 80 to 90 g per serving—a wallop of fat for breakfast that can keep you satisfied all the way through to dinner.

If you are dealing with hunger or food cravings, this nearly always represents a failure to take in sufficient quantities of fats and oils, a virtual "fat deficiency." Whip some coconut oil into your coffee with an immersion blender, drop a big dollop of melted coconut oil into your smoothie, eat the fat on that pork or beef, or slather more organic butter or extra-virgin olive oil over your eggs and vegetables and salads, and cravings will disappear.

You will also rediscover the lost dimensions of flavor added back when you include more fat. Meats taste more flavorful, baked dishes will be richer, even simple eggs cooked in leftover bacon grease will bring "oohs" and "ahhhs." This is one of the main reasons why your unconverted family members, skeptical of or resistant to making the shift to the Wheat Belly lifestyle, will still enjoy the deeper flavors of your cooking.

No Gluten-Free Foods

I've said it before, but it is surprising how many people completely booby-trap their wheat- and grain-free lifestyle by using gluten-free foods made with awful ingredients that shut down any hope of losing weight: cornflour, rice flour, tapioca starch, and potato flour. Gluten-free foods made with these ingredients, in fact, typically cause substantial weight *gain*, as well as a host of other health problems. You can indeed follow a gluten-free lifestyle, but just don't fall for the terrible products sold by unscrupulous food manufacturers smelling a profit opportunity. Absolutely avoid gluten-free foods made with these ingredients.

Keep an Eye on Carbs

While we've discussed this before, it is such a common tripping point that it is worth reiterating. Managing carbs is like managing money: Stay within your budget and everything balances out, and maybe you'll have a little left over at the end of the month for something special; overspend and it's going to hurt.

While carbohydrates and sugars tend to largely manage themselves after wheat and grains have been removed, some people continue to stick to old habits and take in enough carbohydrates to provoke insulin and thereby turn off the capacity to lose weight. This is where an awareness of carbohydrate intake can play a role.

It pays to look at the nutritional content of foods, both processed and unprocessed, as discussed in Chapter 2. Choose a resource—smartphone app, handbook, Web site—that lists the total carbohydrates and fiber in various foods, and perform this simple calculation:

NET CARBS = TOTAL CARBS – FIBER

Do not exceed 15 g net carbs per meal because each time you exceed this value, you trigger insulin that, in turn, turns off your ability to lose weight. Simple habits, such as a glass of orange juice with breakfast or a container of flavored yogurt with lunch, are among the booby-traps that will trigger this weight-loss-blocking effect.

Managing carbohydrates is important even before and during exercise, a confusing point for many people who enjoy casual, or even serious, levels of exercise (see "Don't Booby-Trap Your Health with Exercise Carbs" on page 217).

Is Dairy Getting in the Whey?

Just as carbohydrates trigger insulin, so can some proteins. This insulin-provoking effect is especially powerful with the whey protein of dairy. For this reason, any whey-containing form of dairy turns off the ability to lose weight in many (though not all) people. It has nothing to do with fat or calories, so don't be sidetracked by low-fat or nonfat dairy products; it's the whey.

The only practical way to determine whether this effect is impairing your ability to lose weight is to eliminate all dairy for 4 weeks. If, after stalling at a weight plateau, you suddenly lose, say, 8 pounds, then the whey effect likely applies to you and you will need to avoid dairy products for as long as you desire weight loss. If nothing happens, then it likely does not apply to you.

Cheese is an uncertainty, since most of the whey is removed in the process of cheese making. There is some residual whey that remains, which may be enough to stall your weight-loss efforts. It is therefore best to eliminate cheese, or at least minimize it, during a weight-loss effort.

Avoid Diet Sodas and Soft Drinks

Diet sodas and soft drinks sweetened with aspartame, sucralose, or saccharine, despite lacking calories, are still responsible for weight gain or blocking weight loss. This is likely due to changes in bowel flora that impair insulin responses, the same sorts of changes that grains provoke. If you desire something beyond water, coffee, or tea, see the suggestions for livening up your water in "Herb- and Fruit-Flavored Drinking Waters" on page 153.

Prescription Drugs That Ambush Weight Loss

A number of drugs prescribed to treat common conditions, such as hypertension, allergies, depression, inflammation, and diabetes, block your ability to lose weight. Further, several of these drugs actually cause weight gain, and most doctors fail to inform their patients of such effects.

Among the drugs that block weight loss are:

- Beta-blockers—metoprolol, atenolol, carvedilol, and propranolol
- Antidepressants—amitriptyline (Elavil), nortriptyline (Pamelor), doxepin, paroxetine (Paxil), trazodone, and others
- Steroids such as prednisone and hydrocortisone (but not inhaled or nasal steroids for allergies)
- Antihistamines—diphenhydramine (Benadryl), fexofenadine (Allegra), cetirizine (Zyrtec), cyproheptadine (Periactin), and

others; note that the widely used sleep aid Tylenol PM contains diphenhydramine
- Lyrica for fibromyalgia and pain
- Valproic acid (Depakote) for seizures
- Actos and Avandia for prediabetes and diabetes
- Insulin—injectable insulin can actually be responsible for astounding quantities of weight gain

Obviously, attempts to reduce or eliminate these drugs should be undertaken with the cooperation of your health care provider, as most of these drugs should not just be stopped. Discuss with your doctor how and why you would like to do this. If you encounter resistance or ignorance, or a refusal to discuss or answer questions, find a health care practitioner who will work with you. Don't be surprised if your doctor denies that these drugs block weight loss or cause weight gain, but such associations have been demonstrated repeatedly in clinical trials. And recognize that many of these drugs were unknowingly prescribed to treat the consequences of wheat and grain consumption in the first place, with many conditions receding with your new wheat- and grain-free lifestyle.

Manage Sleep

You have to face a basic health truth: If you compromise on quantity or quality of sleep, you will not lose weight.

Sleep deprivation has numerous health implications beyond just crabbiness and daytime sleepiness. The physiologic disruptions of sleep deprivation include increased risk for high blood pressure, asthma, arthritis, diabetes, heart disease, and stroke. Lack of sleep increases cortisol and insulin, impairs the effects of insulin, and increases appetite, resulting in an increased calorie intake of 300 to 559 calories per day, mostly from snacking. The entire process adds up to stalled weight loss or weight gain. And the less sleep you get, the worse it gets, starting with just a single night of reduced sleep.

Several days per week of lost sleep can therefore yield substantial impact on appetite and calorie intake. If you do the arithmetic, three nights a week of poor sleep can add 22 pounds of weight gain over the course of a year.

How much sleep is enough for overall health and to gain control over weight? It varies from individual to individual, but most people require 7½ hours every night. After several days of reduced sleep, a "sleep debt" accumulates that magnifies the metabolic distortions that contribute to weight gain and unhealthy effects. One night of adequate sleep does not fully pay down the sleep debt. Several days of full sleep beyond the usual 7½ hours may be required to normalize glucose, insulin, and cortisol distortions.

You may have noticed that normal, uninterrupted sleep occurs in 90-minute cycles (e.g., 6 hours, 7½ hours, 9 hours) that allow your brain to cycle through all sleep phases, from light sleep to the deepest phases, including rapid eye movement (REM) sleep filled with dreams. Because it's best to adhere to this normal cycling of sleep, set your clock or alarm to a quantity of time that adheres to this rhythm, as it increases daytime alertness and mood. There are also several devices now available that can waken you gently at the set time using, for instance, increasingly bright light, sound, or vibration. Smartphone apps are also appearing, often coupled to a device (such as the Lark wristband or the UP system by Jawbone) to gently awaken you after tracking your sleep behavior and quality over the preceding night.

Sometimes, a little help may be necessary to reestablish healthy sleep habits. Useful natural sleep aids include:

MELATONIN. Melatonin is the natural hormone of sleep and circadian rhythms, its release activated with dark and inhibited with light. (Sleeping in complete darkness, with no exposure to a bathroom light when going to the bathroom, for instance, is a natural way to increase melatonin release.) It is not a sleeping pill; it is a sleep hormone, simply making your body more receptive to sleep. Melatonin supplementation can hasten the onset of sleep, make sleep deeper, and discourage early awakening. It also has substantial effects in reducing blood pressure, especially when taken as a sustained-release preparation. Melatonin is not habit forming and has proven safe, even with extended use.

People who have tried melatonin often declare that it doesn't work, but a little finesse in its use can go a long way in obtaining the desired effect. If difficulty falling asleep is the problem, take it approximately 2 or 3 hours before the desired bedtime. If staying asleep is your struggle, then taking it right at bedtime may work better to discourage early awakening; consider a time-release preparation for sustained effect. It also helps to experiment with different doses. While some people have wonderfully restful sleep with just 0.5 mg, others require 3, 5, 10, even 20 mg to obtain the same effect.

TRYPTOPHAN. Taken at doses in increments of 500 mg (e.g., 1,000, 1,500, 2,000, 2,500, 3,000 mg), the amino acid tryptophan enhances sleep. Supplementation increases brain serotonin and melatonin, which benefits sleep at night and mood during the day. Tryptophan can be taken by itself or in combination with melatonin and tends to not leave any residual effect upon awakening. Tryptophan should not be used if you are taking certain antidepressant medication, as excessive levels of serotonin can result.

PREBIOTIC FIBERS/RESISTANT STARCHES. Yes, the fiber strategies discussed in Chapter 4 and incorporated into the Detox Shakes that add wonderfully to your overall health recovery also enhance sleep. By taking their fibers before bedtime, some people experience deeper, more restful sleep filled with vivid dreams. This is a great time to use inulin powder, fructooligosaccharides, or other products (see Appendix B), rather than a gut-busting Detox Shake, to avoid going to bed with a full stomach. Many people describe some pretty wild and entertainingly creative dreams following this strategy.

Thyroid Chaos

Like the speed dial on your blender, the thyroid controls the "speed" of your metabolism. Too high and you lose weight despite eating like a horse. Too low and no matter how meticulous your diet or how many calories you cut back, you fail to lose weight or gain weight. Just right and your efforts are rewarded by natural weight loss when nutrition is managed properly. Thyroid dysfunction sufficient to impair weight loss is, unfortunately, very common, much of it initiated by wheat and grains (though not entirely reversed with their removal), as well as other causes. Thyroid issues are often undiagnosed, underappreciated, and misunderstood by doctors.

About 20 percent of people starting the Wheat Belly 10-Day Detox are deficient in iodine, the trace mineral required by the thyroid gland to produce thyroid hormones. This is why iodine is included in the list of essential strategies to add after wheat and grain elimination discussed in Chapter 4. If iodine is the cause for failed weight loss, as well as hypothyroid symptoms such as cold hands and feet, hair loss, and low energy, then iodine supplementation is the fix. (The only people who should not take iodine on their own are those with a history of autoimmune thyroid disease; see the cautions discussed in Chapter 4.) For many people, though, there is more to the thyroid question than iodine.

Of all endocrine glands, the thyroid gland is the most susceptible to autoimmune damage, i.e., damage from your immune system that misguidedly attacks it and impairs its production of thyroid hormone. The most common trigger of autoimmune thyroid diseases such as Hashimoto's thyroiditis? The gliadin protein of wheat and related proteins of other grains. Getting rid of wheat and grains therefore removes the trigger for autoimmune thyroid damage in the majority. But the vulnerable and delicate thyroid gland and its production of thyroid hormones typically do not recover from the beating, and prescription thyroid hormones are usually still necessary, even long after autoimmune inflammation has subsided.

The problems with thyroid health are worse than that of just iodine deficiency and grains. We live during a peculiar era, a time when industrial compounds have proliferated to such an extraordinary degree that everyone is exposed to chemicals that disrupt the network of hormonal signals that determine thyroid status—a form of endocrine disruption. Disruption can occur at the brain level (hypothalamus and pituitary that control the thyroid), at the thyroid gland level, or even at the level of tissues, such as fat cells, liver, and muscle, dependent on thyroid hormones. Thyroid disruption can originate with perfluorooctanoic acid residues from Teflon in your cooking, restaurant food, or groundwater. It can be caused by triclosan in antibacterial hand soaps and hand sanitizers. It can be due to polybrominated diphenyl ethers from the flame retardant in carpeting. There are hundreds more.

If visceral fat is present in the tummy, then this unique fat also disrupts thyroid function due to the flood of inflammatory proteins it releases that interfere with the function of thyroid hormones. This can occur with or without interference of thyroid function by autoimmune inflammation.

In other words, thyroid dysfunction sufficient to impair weight loss is common. But there is yet another problem in this tangle of thyroid issues: Most doctors are unaware of the above issues, unaware that the old rules for diagnosing thyroid dysfunction no longer apply due to disruption by industrial chemicals. It means that, even if doctors manage to diagnose hypothyroidism (low levels of thyroid hormone), they will only prescribe the T4 thyroid hormone but neglect to address T3, the truly active form of thyroid hormone. This results in someone taking T4 as levo-thyroxine (Synthroid), being told that their thyroid status is fine, yet continuing to struggle with hypothyroid symptoms such as weight gain, cold hands and feet, hair loss, even increased cardio-vascular risk due to disruption of T3 function or blocked conver-sion of T4 to T3 (how most T3 in the body is produced).

The key is to identify a health care practitioner who is enlightened on thyroid issues if you have such symptoms or if you have been prescribed T4 without T3. Look for a functional medicine practitioner, a naturopath, or someone who uses a compounding pharmacy to mix individualized thyroid prescrip-tions (ask the pharmacist at a compounding pharmacy in your area, one that is licensed to mix its own individualized prescrip-tions). The solution is usually as easy as replacing the T4 with a T4/T3 combination preparation (such as Armour Thyroid or Nature-Throid) or adding T3 (as liothyronine or Cytomel). The restraint on weight loss from thyroid dysfunction will be released.

The Weight Booby-Trap of Emotional Stress

When you are stressed, the stress hormone cortisol is released at higher-than-normal levels. This can be like taking the cortisol-like drug prednisone, which is often prescribed to reduce inflam-mation and results in dramatic weight gain. A course of prednisone prescribed for a few weeks for an asthma attack, for instance, can result in 10 to 20 pounds of weight gain in that short period.

If you are under prolonged and substantial stress, high levels of cortisol can make it virtually impossible for you to lose weight. The fix for this issue may not be easy, as it means finding ways to

NICOLE, 48, flight attendant, Georgia

"On Day 1, I felt good. It was a little overwhelming at the grocery store, and I had to visit two different stores to get what I needed. On Day 2, I developed a low-grade headache by evening time. By Day 3, the headache was still low grade but semi-bearable. Twice the headache mutated into a full-on migraine. I was moving a lot slower than I usually do throughout the day. There was an element of fogginess in my daily routine that I couldn't seem to shake. On the morning of Day 4, I woke up with heartburn and a queasy stomach. I found it hard to eat anything, as nothing was appealing, but, by the evening, I was hungry and a bit more energetic. The most bothersome symptom was the constant runny nose. I didn't travel anywhere without a pack of tissues.

"By Day 5, I felt much, much better and even had the urge to exercise, although I won't—doctor's orders! My energy today is the most it's been in 5 days. My headache is gone completely, and I am thinking clearer and more focused. The most positive effect for me was that my work uniform was looser. I've always slept well, but now I find that I sleep longer. I have also noticed that I don't feel like I'm in a fog. I think clearer and am more focused. I definitely have a lot more energy."

By the end of her 10-day detox experience, Nicole had lost 6.4 pounds, or 3.4 percent of her starting body weight.

deal with the stress. I recognize that it is not always easy to accomplish this if, for example, stress originates with caring for an aging parent, an impaired child, an unhappy marriage, or other situation that you cannot easily brush off or walk away from. In many such situations, there are no quick and easy fixes. The solution involves finding ways to manage the stress to try to reduce the physiological toll it's exacting on your body. It will involve solutions that require ongoing, long-term effort such as exercise, the companionship of friends and family, counseling, yoga, meditation, biofeedback, and getting time away from the source of stress, if possible.

Don't Booby-Trap Your Health with Exercise Carbs

Here's a common tripping point: Someone who likes to exercise by jogging several miles or engaging in aerobic exercise for prolonged periods (with, say, jazzercise or Zumba) will say, "I need to load up on carbohydrates before exercise to have energy." Or they adhere to the habit of carrying an "energy bar" or other sugar/carbohydrate source to ensure sustained energy levels during exercise. Or they use some form of high-carb "recovery" drink or food after finishing. All of these strategies turn off your ability to lose weight and have adverse consequences for long-term health. This is true for the casual exerciser as well as for elite athletes who are training for a marathon, triathlon, or other sustained endurance effort. It applies to everybody. Carb loading or exercise carbs are not only unnecessary, they are harmful; eventually, the harmful effects will catch up to them, despite the healthy practice of exercise.

One of the goals of engaging in the 10-day detox, as well as the long-term Wheat Belly lifestyle, is to become less reliant on the sugar stored in your liver as glycogen for energy. Glycogen is the lengthy chain of sugars that can be "burned" for energy on demand, such as during exercise. The average person has no more than around 40 minutes' worth of energy stored as glycogen in the liver. Once it's depleted by biking vigorously for 12 miles, for example, a dramatic drop in energy will be encountered, which some call hitting the wall or the bonk.

Conventional "wisdom" is to therefore load up on carbohydrates and sugars ahead of the effort (thus the pasta dinners traditionally held the night before a marathon) or to carry ripe bananas, energy gels, sports drinks or bars, or other commercial products created for this purpose. While these strategies do indeed work to provide a constant flow of sugar to replenish liver glycogen, they also result in surges in blood sugar to high levels, as well as an osmotic effect (pulling water into the intestines) from the plentiful sugar in the gut. This is why there are so many portable toilets along the marathon route and people experience vomiting and diarrhea with their efforts. It also keeps you dependent on a constant flow of sugars to replenish liver glycogen, while turning off the capacity to draw energy from stored fat.

A better solution consistent with the Wheat Belly lifestyle that will enhance health and not impair your ability to lose weight: Avoid all such sugary products before and during exercise. This approach works only if you have engaged in the Wheat Belly lifestyle of consuming no grains or sugars, have limited carbohydrates to no more than 15 g net per meal, and have endured your detoxification/withdrawal process and then waited an additional 4 to 6 weeks. This last component of waiting a month or longer represents the time required for your body to convert from relying on liver glycogen as a primary source of energy to fat mobilizing for energy. In other words, while your liver contains energy sufficient to sustain around 40 minutes of vigorous physical effort, energy stored as fat—even on a slender person—is sufficient to provide energy for weeks. High-performing athletes therefore should be burning fat, not liver glycogen. (Doesn't it make more sense to draw off the considerable energy in your body stored as fat? That's how humans have done it for millions of years—they didn't have energy products to fuel their hunt for dinner—and that's how healthy modern humans should do it.)

A few of our detox panelists fell into this trap, observing that they "needed" to load up on some carbohydrate/sugar source prior to or during exercise in order to perform. Do not give in to this. Accept that your running, biking, or other performance will be impaired during the 4- to 6-week period. But once that period is over, your exercise performance will match or even exceed the level you'd achieved before engaging in this lifestyle—that's when you'll know that your body has successfully made the transition.

The only time I have seen that some form of carbohydrate or sugar *might* be helpful is during extreme endurance efforts, such as mile 14 of a marathon, mile 50 of a biking trip, or a similar intensive, long-term effort—but never for an hour of dancing or a 3-mile run. Even with extreme endurance, only a modest quantity of sugar is required in the midst of the effort, such as 25 g in the form of a banana or a sip of a sports drink, to maintain energy. This concept of sustained low-carb performance is catching on among a greater number of elite athletes, and more of them are observing that they need only water and electrolytes to fuel their effort, not carbohydrates or sugars.

Am I Too Skinny?

Yes, it happens. In the midst of the worst epidemic of obesity ever witnessed in the history of mankind, there are people who (1) don't want to lose weight yet desire the health benefits of the Wheat Belly lifestyle, or (2) have already achieved their desired weight and want the weight loss to stop. This is, of course, not an issue for most people during their 10-day detox, but it can become a question in the coming months. Should this question arise, consider the following:

ARE YOU REALLY TOO SKINNY? Or are you normal but just look too skinny in a world of overweight and obese people? Don't laugh: It's actually quite common on this lifestyle. Take a look at an old movie from the 1950s, for instance, and notice that Doris Day, Lucille Ball, Spencer Tracy, and everyone else is "skinny," just like you. They are normal. Many people who believe they are too slender have really just lost perspective because of the peculiar times we live in. And don't believe the people around you who practice the principle of "misery loves company" and might try to convince you that, because you no longer look like them, you are unhealthy or unacceptably thin. You're normal, and you should be proud of it.

DON'T LIMIT CALORIES. The Wheat Belly approach does not limit calories, fat, or protein. You will not find a single word in this book telling you to cut back on calories, even if you have 100 pounds to lose. We don't count points or push the plate away or use smaller plates and bowls, etc. If you feel that you have lost too much weight, eat more avocados, more coconut oil, more fat on your meat or poultry, and more raw nuts. Go back for seconds and ignore all the envious looks.

ADD BACK MUSCLE. Weight loss is unavoidably a combination of fat loss and muscle loss. If you lose 30 pounds in total weight, 10 pounds of that lost weight is typically muscle. (In my experience, following the Wheat Belly lifestyle results in less muscle loss than with typical diet plans, but it still happens to some degree.) The muscle is easily regained through strength training. Concentrate on rebuilding large muscles, such as your thighs, chest, shoulders, and upper back, for best effect. You don't have to be muscle-bound; just regain lost muscle by devoting 15 to 20 minutes twice per week to some form of strength-training exercises.

Take comfort in the fact that, minus the appetite stimulant in modern wheat and related grains, most people gravitate back toward a healthy weight. Modest adjustments in perception, diet, and exercise might be necessary, but you will not—provided you are eating real, single-ingredient healthy foods and not sweating calories—become emaciated and disappear into a pile of dust.

PINCH YOURSELF

By now, I hope that you begin to understand that so much of what you had come to believe about health and nutrition was really just awful advice, the misguided beliefs of health care practitioners, bad science and misinterpretation, or just plain dishonesty and deceptive marketing. Once you hear the truth, a lot of things begin to make sense, and many missing pieces fall into place. No, you are not overweight due to sloth and gluttony. No, you are not taking multiple prescription medications because of bad genes and bad luck. No, you are not feeling awful with pain and swelling while aging rapidly because of some mysterious illness that no doctor has been able to diagnose. No, the ideas of a "balanced diet" and "everything in moderation" and "just a little bit won't hurt" are not recipes for success. But now you know.

I hope that the information you've encountered through the Wheat Belly 10-Day Detox has enlightened you, much like shining a bright light into a dark room you were trying to navigate, blind and helpless. You finally are empowered to take back control over so many aspects of health and weight—slender, flexible, happy, pain-free, likely drug-free, and looking like you turned back the clock 10 or more years in the process.

CHAPTER

9

AFTER THE DETOX: GRAIN-FREE AND REBORN

CONGRATULATIONS: YOU SURVIVED—detoxified, empowered, and emboldened! I confidently predict that there is a spectacular future ahead for you, likely very different from the one you may have been anticipating just 10 days ago.

By now, you have reorganized your kitchen to be confidently grain-free; shopped, cooked, and eaten your way through the menu plan; added the essential nutritional supplements and prebiotic fibers; and are starting to feel really terrific. You may be well on your way to reducing or eliminating prescription drugs or obtaining relief from joint pain, gastrointestinal turmoil, skin rashes, headaches, or other health struggles. Perhaps you've baked a dish or two that have begun converting your family to this new and healthy way of living.

I hope that the changes are becoming so visible and obvious that friends and family are sneaking admiring glances at you, wondering just what you are doing to look so good. Surely you snuck away for a quick tummy-tuck, round of liposuction, and face-lift! But you know better, understanding that it is the detoxification from a potent and ubiquitous dietary disrupter that has permitted your body to undergo changes that are far better and healthier than the crude and superficial results achieved through such procedures.

Now it's time to continue what you've started and enjoy your rebirth—I don't believe it is an exaggeration to call it that—taking your new journey of amazing health, performance, and appearance to higher levels that were not possible before your detox experience. It's also time to set the example for others, so that they learn your new health, vigor, and youth were no accident or the handiwork of some skillful plastic surgeon; it was the result of setting diet right.

You have learned that the wheat and grain detoxification process is most certainly not a matter of cutting carbs or calories. The Wheat Belly lifestyle succeeds on such a grand scale because we are detoxifying from a dietary poison. Just as the destructive effects of cigarette smoking can only begin to be reversed by not smoking cigarettes, so the body cannot begin its healing process unless the grains that taste so good but hurt so bad are removed. Wheat and grain elimination, followed by the correction of all residual abnormalities, is in many ways bigger than quitting cigarettes, as it touches such diverse aspects of life and health.

Yes, by eliminating the foods that we are told over and over again should dominate every meal, we experience benefits for health and weight that are unmatched by any weight-loss program, exercise, nutritional supplement, or drug, even outdoing the benefits of such awful practices as inserting a gastric band or undergoing gastric bypass surgery. And, yes, you had to spend a bit more on your grocery bill to restock your kitchen with a new set of ingredients, but think of what you will save by not having to take two, three, or 10 prescription drugs, not having to take anti-inflammatory and pain medications day after day, and not having to be hospitalized and subjected to medical procedures. So I see wonderful things ahead for both your health and financial life, as you will be spared the crippling health costs that burden so many people as they age, as a result of eating all those "healthy whole grains."

Are you also beginning to grasp the magnitude of the blunder we've made as a society in incorporating wheat and grains into the human diet? To make matters worse, agribusiness magnified their destructive health impact by introducing some extreme changes for its own purposes. Then, doubly worse, we are advised that wheat and grains should dominate our diets and be the go-to foods for every meal, 7 days a week, 365 days a year, while food manufacturers packed grains into virtually every processed food. We may not ever get the USDA, other agencies, or Big Food to admit to their enormous mistake, but we don't have to wait for them to own up: We can just take on this dietary correction ourselves and enjoy the tremendous health benefits that follow.

I truly mean it when I say that, after you complete this 10-day detoxification process, you will begin to think about your life as "before Wheat Belly" and the "rebirth after Wheat Belly." I am often astounded at just how much misery people endure for decades until they discover that the pain, suffering, ceaseless hunger, and "need" for medical care all began with the innocent bagel for breakfast, whole grain sandwich for lunch, or pasta for dinner. But this 10-day experience has begun the process to undo all of it, starting you on a new chapter of life and health.

The detox process was intended to get you started on the right path. Unlike other detoxes that end with whatever detox strategy was involved, this detoxification requires that you stay away from the toxic source—wheat and grains—for a lifetime. For the rebirth of ideal health, I would also encourage you to continue the nutritional supplement program and eating style that you learned about throughout this process.

I'd therefore like to close with a challenge. Now that you have accomplished this entire starting process, I would challenge you to continue it for a lifetime. I would like to hear that you have gotten healthier and stronger, that you have achieved your weight-loss goal, and that you have reversed most, if not all, health conditions that you endured during your wheat- and grain-consuming days while shortening the list of medications or eliminating them entirely. I would also like to hear that you look and feel like you haven't looked and felt in decades, serving as an inspiration for people around you who cannot get over your transformation. I want to hear that people cannot believe you are 55 years old because you don't look a day over 35. I challenge you to continue the momentum you've built up in this 10-day process to take your health even further.

Should you desire more support and resources to stay on course, start by engaging in the conversations on the Wheat Belly Facebook page (facebook.com/OfficialWheatBelly), where you can relate your detox experience along the way, ask questions, share food and recipe ideas, and post your stories and photos of success. Even as a newcomer, you will learn that everyone loves hearing about new successes or coming to your assistance with help and suggestions. You will see that you are far from alone in this experience; you'll be part of an international movement to take back health and share in a powerful and enlightening life-style now followed by people on every continent. Our shared experiences in reversing the crippling effects of conventional advice to eat wheat and grains bind this community together, along with an eagerness to help cultivate this message. By participating in these conversations, you will recognize that you have become part of a large community of people who are enjoying impressive levels of health, day-to-day functioning, and physical performance. You will find it engaging, enlightening, and endlessly entertaining.

If you desire additional recipes, see the *Wheat Belly Cookbook* and *Wheat Belly 30-Minute (or Less!) Cookbook*. And, if you are looking to take health several steps higher, including further undoing complex health conditions or further trimming your reliance on medications, as well as gaining better understanding about a wealth of other health issues, see *Wheat Belly Total Health*.

Imagine your children and your children's children learning about this message of empowerment early in life—and being spared all the weight and health problems that you have suffered for decades, not having to submit to medical testing, not needing all the prescription drugs, and not having to endure all manner of symptoms as you may have done for many years. I hope that you use the lessons learned through this detox process as the launching pad to bring change to your own life over many more years, as well as to the lives around you.

Now go have some cheesecake!

APPENDIX A

Wheat Belly Detox Shopping List

IF YOU WERE to equip your kitchen with just about everything you needed to create the recipes in the Wheat Belly 10-Day Detox Menu Plan, as well as other dishes that fit into a Wheat Belly lifestyle, this is what it would contain. I would not advise you to use this as an actual shopping list, however, as not all ingredients are used in the 10-Day Menu Plan; they are included more as a reference to determine whether an ingredient fits into this life-style or not.

Your shopping list, the one you actually bring with you to the grocery store as you proceed through the detox, is best compiled on the day(s) when or immediately preceding the day you will actually make the dishes, to ensure freshness of your ingredients. The day-by-day shopping list follows this more comprehensive list.

Almond milk, unsweetened

Baking powder

Bicarbonate of soda

Cauliflower

Cheeses (preferably full-fat, organic)

Chia seeds

Chocolate—100% chocolate, 85% cacao or greater

Chocolate chips, dark

Cocoa powder, unsweetened

Coconut, shredded and unsweetened; coconut flakes

Coconut flour

Coconut milk—canned for thickness; carton for drinking

Courgettes

Dried fruit, unsweetened

Extracts—natural almond, coconut, vanilla, and peppermint

Flaxseeds, preferably ground golden

Ground almonds/flour

Ground nuts—ground pecans, walnuts, hazelnuts

Inulin powder

Nut and seed butters—almond butter, peanut butter, sunflower seed butter

Nuts—raw almonds, pecans, walnuts, pistachios, hazelnuts, Brazil nuts; chopped walnuts or pecans for baking

Oils—extra-virgin olive, coconut, organic butter, ghee, avocado, flaxseed, walnut, extra-light olive, nonhydrogenated lard or tallow

Seeds—raw sunflower, raw pumpkin, sesame, and chia

Shirataki noodles (in the refrigerated section)

Spaghetti squash

Sweeteners—liquid stevia, powdered stevia (pure or with inulin, not maltodextrin), monk fruit, powdered erythritol, xylitol

10-DAY MENU PLAN DAY-BY-DAY SHOPPING LIST

Here are the ingredients required if you adhere to the 10-Day Menu Plan as written. Obviously, to save time and effort, shop for several days at a time. The ingredients that are used repeatedly or in more than one recipe are listed at the top as "Frequently Used

Ingredients." Each day's shopping list assumes that you have already purchased the frequently used ingredients and that your kitchen is already stocked with common items such as eggs and ground pepper.

Be prepared for greater up-front costs as you discard grain products and restock your kitchen with grain-free, healthy ingredients. Once you stock your shelves and refrigerator and accumulate all the tools you need, the costs will drop.

Frequently Used Ingredients

Ingredients for Detox Shakes—white potatoes, green bananas, inulin powder, unsweetened coconut/almond/hemp milk, coconut oil, raw pumpkin seeds, stevia drops or your choice of safe sweetener, as well as the ingredients for each unique shake (e.g., unsweetened cocoa powder, unsweetened apple purée, unsweetened pineapple chunks)

Coconut oil

Extra-virgin olive oil

Butter, organic

Vinegar—white, apple cider, balsamic

Hot-pepper sauce

Mayonnaise

Gluten-free soy sauce or tamari

Vanilla extract

Almond extract

Coconut milk, canned

Onions

Garlic cloves

Parmesan or Romano cheese, grated

Raw sunflower seeds

Raw pumpkin seeds

Raw almonds, sliced

Raw pecans, chopped or whole

Raw walnuts, chopped or whole

Shredded unsweetened coconut

Ground almonds/flour

Ground golden flaxseeds

Coconut flour

Curry powder

Ground ginger

Onion powder

Ground cinnamon

Ground cloves

Ground nutmeg

Dried rosemary

Dried basil

Dried oregano

Garlic powder

Sea salt

Sweetener—your choice of liquid stevia, powdered stevia, monk fruit, erythritol, xylitol, inulin, Truvía, Swerve, Wheat-Free Market Foods Sweetener

DAY 1

Apricot Ginger "Granola"—dried apricots (5), allspice

Cream of Broccoli Soup—chicken stock (1 litre), broccoli (450 g/1 lb)

Italian Sausage and Pepper Pizza—shredded mozzarella cheese (300 g/11 oz), Italian sausages (loose or in casing, 225g/8 oz), red pepper (1), green or yellow pepper (1), pizza sauce (1 cup), crushed red chillies

DAY 2

Berry Coconut Quick Muffin—fresh or frozen mixed berries (55 g/2 oz)

Wheat Belly Herbed Focaccia Bread—shredded mozzarella cheese (150 g/5 oz), black or kalamata olives (80 g/3 oz), sun-dried tomatoes (40 g/1½ oz, preferably in oil)

Aubergine Lasagna—aubergines (2 medium), tomato (marinara) sauce (2 × 375 g/13 oz jars), fresh or dried basil, fresh or dried oregano, ricotta cheese (450 g/1 lb), mozzarella cheese (450 g/1 lb)

DAY 3

Mediterranean "Pasta" Salad—courgettes (450 g/1 lb), cherry tomatoes (225 g/8 oz), cucumber (1 medium), spring onions (5–6), black or kalamata olives (80 g/3oz), pepperoni (225 g/8 oz), fresh or dried basil, fresh or dried oregano

Bacon-Topped Meat Loaf with Mushrooms and Gravy—minced beef (450 g/1 lb), minced pork (450 g/1 lb), carrots (310 g/11 oz shredded), green pepper (1), bacon (4 rashers), button mushrooms (110 g/4 oz), beef stock (240 ml/8 fl oz)

Mashed "Potatoes"—cauliflower (1 large head)

DAY 4

Spicy Italian Frittata—Italian sausages (225 g/8 oz loose or in casing), spinach or kale (60 g/2½ oz), red pepper (1)

Spaghetti with Meatballs—minced beef (700 g/1½ lb), fresh or dried basil, fresh or dried oregano, courgettes (700 g/1½ lb), tomato sauce (2 × 400 g/14 oz)

DAY 5

Curried Chicken Soup—chicken breasts (450 g/1 lb), shiitake mushrooms (110 g /4 oz), chicken stock (1 litre), coriander (2 tablespoons chopped)

Fettucine Alfredo—courgettes (900 g/2 lb), double cream or canned coconut milk (120 ml/4 fl oz)

Chocolate Avocado Pudding—avocados (3 large ripe), unsweetened cocoa powder (60 g/2½ oz), optional fresh berries (110 g/4 oz)

DAY 6

Aubergine Mini Pizzas—aubergine (1 medium), pizza sauce (250 g/9 oz), pepperoni (50 g/2 oz), shredded mozzarella cheese (35 g/1 oz)

Pork Thai Stir-Fry—spring onions (4–5), pork (your choice of cut, e.g., pork chop, loin, ham; 450 g/1 lb), fresh ginger (1 tablespoon grated), broccoli (1 large head), shiitake mushrooms (110 g/4 oz), red curry sauce (1 tablespoon), fish sauce (60 ml/2 fl oz), coriander (2 tablespoons chopped)

DAY 7

Chorizo, Pepper, and Avocado Fry-Up—radishes (450 g 1 lb), spring onions (4), chorizo sausage (350 g/12 oz), green pepper (1), kale or spinach (60 g/2½ oz), avocado (1 large)

Bacon-Wrapped Chicken Breasts Stuffed with Spinach, Mushrooms, and Roasted Red Peppers—chicken breasts (4 breasts, about 900 g/2 lb), portobello mushrooms (110 g/4 oz), roasted red peppers (170 g/6 oz), spinach (120 g/4 oz fresh or 275 g/10 oz frozen), bacon (8 rashers)

DAY 8

Spicy Minestrone—chicken stock (1 litre), chopped tomatoes (400 g/14 oz can), tomato purée (175 g/6 oz can), celery (2 sticks), green beans (225 g/8 oz), pinto beans (425 g/15 oz can), button mushrooms (110 g/4 oz), spinach (120 g/4 oz chopped fresh or 275 g/10 oz frozen chopped), fresh basil (15 g/½ oz)

Prawn Fried "Rice"—cauliflower (1 head), spring onions (5–6), prawns (450 g/1 lb cooked), fresh ginger (1 tablespoon grated), carrots (155 g/5½ oz grated), green pepper (1), fish sauce (2 tablespoons), sesame oil (2 tablespoons)

DAY 9

Jumbo Gingerbread Nut Muffins—all ingredients are in the Frequently Used Ingredients list

Bratwurst with Peppers and Sauerkraut—caraway seeds (1 teaspoon), celery seeds (½ teaspoon), bratwurst or other spicy sausage (450 g/1 lb), green peppers (2), sauerkraut (300 g/11 oz)

"Potato" Salad—turnips (900 g/2 lb), white onion (1), dill pickles (2), Dijon mustard (2 teaspoons), paprika (1 teaspoon)

DAY 10

BLT Wrap—lettuce or spinach (20 g/¾ oz), bacon
(2 rashers), tomato (1)

Roasted Brussels Sprouts and Ham Fry-Up—Brussels
sprouts (450 g/1 lb), portobello mushrooms (110g/4 oz),
sweet potato (1 medium), ham (precooked, 350 g/12 oz)

KITCHEN DEVICES

- A spiral-cutting device to create "spaghetti" from courgettes, such as Spirelli, a spiralizer, Veggetti, the Benriner Spiral Cutter, or the Sur La Table Vegetable and Fruit Spiral Slicer.

- A grinding device: While a food processor works great to grind nuts and other foods, cleanup can be a hassle. I use a simple food chopper (KitchenAid sells one, among others) to grind efficiently with quick cleanup. Even a coffee grinder can get the job done with less cleanup.

- A powerful blender: It helps to have a blender with a motor powerful enough to not stall when we make our Wheat Belly Detox Shakes, which include ingredients like a coarsely chopped potato or green banana. A Vitamix handles these ingredients easily. I also used a less powerful NutriBullet, which handled the job without problems.

- Parchment paper: Grain-free baking involves less hassle with quicker cleanup if you use parchment paper to bake pizzas and other dishes.

APPENDIX B

Additional Resources

RECOGNIZE HIDDEN SOURCES OF WHEAT AND GRAINS

You will see from the following lists that grains come in an incredible variety of forms, often hidden as some additive, thickener, or coating. The variety of colorful names can falsely lull you into thinking that no wheat is present: couscous, matzo, orzo, graham, faro, panko, and bran, for example. But all are wheat. A similar situation applies to corn.

Be aware of the potential for grain contamination from utensils, airborne particles, or liquids. Cross-contamination is most problematic for people with extreme gluten sensitivities or an allergy to a grain component. If a food is labeled "gluten-free," then it should have been prepared in a facility where cross-contamination would not have occurred. Very few restaurants have the ability to avoid cross-contamination, though an increasing number are taking on the challenge as the market for these foods grows.

To qualify as "gluten-free" according to FDA criteria, products must be both free of gluten and produced in a gluten-free facility. The FDA's cutoff for qualifying as gluten-free is that the food should contain no more than 20 parts per million. This means that, for the seriously sensitive, even an ingredient label that does not list wheat or any buzzwords for wheat such as "modified food starch" can still contain some measure of gluten. When in doubt, contact the customer service department for the product to inquire whether a gluten-free facility was used. More and more manufacturers are starting to specify whether products are gluten-free or not gluten-free on their Web sites.

Note that "wheat-free" does not equate with "gluten-free" in food labeling. "Wheat-free" can mean, for instance, that barley malt or rye is used in place of wheat, but both are sources of gluten and other grain-sourced contaminants. Also recognize that, even though corn products are often used in gluten-free foods, the zein protein of corn can mimic many of the effects of the gliadin protein of wheat; we therefore avoid all sources of corn.

Here are some not-so-obvious foods that can contain wheat, as well as some wheat-based ingredients in foods that might appear benign. A question mark (?) following an item means it is either variable (some products contain wheat while others do not) or uncertain (given manufacturers' reluctance or inability to specify the source).

Hidden Sources of Wheat

Baguette

Beignet

Bran

Brioche

Bulgur

Burrito

Caramel coloring (?)

Caramel flavoring (?)

Couscous

Crepe

Croutons

Dextrimaltose

Durum

Einkorn

Emmer

Emulsifiers

Farina

Faro

Focaccia

Fu (gluten in Asian foods)

Gnocchi

Graham flour

Gravy

Hydrolyzed vegetable protein

Hydrolyzed wheat starch

Kamut

Maltodextrin

Matzo

Modified food starch (?)

Orzo

Panko (a bread crumb mixture used in Japanese cooking)

Ramen

Roux (wheat-based sauce or thickener)

Rusk

Rye

Seitan (nearly pure gluten used in place of meat)

Semolina

Soba (mostly buckwheat but usually also includes wheat)

Spelt

Stabilizers

Strudel

Tabbouleh

Tart

Textured vegetable protein (?)

Triticale

Triticum

Udon

Vital wheat gluten

Wheat bran

Wheat germ

Wraps

Hidden Sources of Corn

Identifying sources of corn is also not always so straightforward. While foods like corn on the cob, cornmeal, high-fructose corn syrup, and popcorn are obvious, there are also many hidden or nonobvious sources of corn.

One of the difficulties with corn products is that, in addition to the above sources, there are literally hundreds of common food ingredients derived from corn—such as dextrose, dextrin, malto-dextrin, high-fructose corn syrup, fructose, maltitol, polydextrose, ethanol, caramel coloring, and artificial flavorings—that will not be identified as being sourced from corn. However, the process to generate these products from corn reduces protein content to negligible levels, and they are therefore generally not a problem for grain exposure for the majority (though these products, especially sugars, pose other problems of their own). Also note that many medications and nutritional supplements contain wheat or corn.

Because of the many ways that corn-derived ingredients can make their way into processed foods, the best policy for the ultra-sensitive is to avoid processed foods as much as possible. Be aware of the potential of corn-derived ingredients if there is suspicion of ongoing exposures.

Among the most common hidden ingredients from corn are:

Grits

Hominy

Hydrolyzed corn protein

Hydrolyzed cornflour

Maize

Mixed vegetable oil, vegetable oil

Modified food starch

Polenta

Zea mays

Zein

SAFE PREMIXED SWEETENER COMBINATIONS

- Truvía—Available widely in major supermarkets, Truvía is a combination of rebiana, an isolate from stevia with less bitterness, and erythritol. Though the erythritol is sourced from corn, which we try to avoid, the corn protein residues are negligible.

- Swerve—This is a combination of erythritol and inulin. The inulin can act as a prebiotic fiber to feed bowel flora.

- Wheat-Free Market Foods Sweetener—This unique combination of monk fruit and erythritol has, teaspoon for teaspoon, four times the sweetness of sugar, allowing a little to go a long way.

IDENTIFYING PROBLEM INGREDIENTS IN PRESCRIPTION DRUGS

If you can obtain the package insert for a prescription drug from the pharmacist or examine the ingredients listed on the package for an over-the-counter drug, you can check for wheat/grain components. You can try just asking the pharmacist, but you likely won't get a helpful answer. Likewise, most doctors do not know what drugs contain grains or gluten in some form.

You can contact the manufacturer of the drug, though this can yield a tangle of uncertainty and the possibility of being bounced around from person to person. It can occasionally yield a straight answer, however, and is worth a try if the package insert or package is unavailable or unhelpful.

There is a Web site where a fairly comprehensive list of gluten-free drugs is maintained by a pharmacist: glutenfreedrugs.com.

SAFELY NAVIGATING ALCOHOLIC BEVERAGES

Provided you choose your sources wisely and drink responsibly, there is no reason alcoholic beverages cannot be a part of your grain-free lifestyle. Making the wrong choice can block weight loss, cause dreaded reexposure reactions to grains (e.g., bloating, diarrhea, joint pain), and even provoke the return of autoimmune conditions that, as you now know, can provoke misery that lasts for weeks to months. On the other hand, choosing alcoholic beverages wisely can mean spending an evening with friends without any such problems. Also bear in mind that, during your 10-day initiation to this lifestyle, any more than one drink per day will turn off that day's capacity for weight loss. So go very lightly or abstain altogether during the detox period or while you are actively trying to lose weight.

Wine

Wine is as close to a near perfect wheat- and gluten-free choice as we get. Combined with the probable health effects that derive from light wine drinking (no more than two 115 ml (4 fl oz) glasses per day), it should be your first choice. Most benefits derive from the dry red wines, less so white, so choose cabernets, merlots, zinfandels, and other dry reds for the benefits as well as the pleasure. Note that wine coolers typically contain barley malt, as well as greater carbohydrate and sugar levels. For these reasons, wine coolers should be avoided.

Beer and Ale

Nearly all ales, beers, malt liquors, and lagers are brewed from grains and are therefore off the list, as there are grain protein residues present—generally 1 to 2 g per 350ml (12 fl oz), enough to stimulate appetite, provoke inflammation, and initiate autoimmunity. People with celiac disease or the most extreme forms of gluten sensitivity should avoid beers altogether except those designated gluten-free. If they're gluten-free, no gliadin or gluten should be present (at least below 20 parts per million, the official American FDA cutoff), but be aware that there remains potential for uncertain reactions from other grain proteins. Those of us without celiac disease or gluten sensitivity seem to do okay with beers brewed from sorghum and rice, but because these also include barley malt, you may have to make your decision on an individual basis. (If a sorghum-based beer causes bloating or abdominal discomfort, for example, you'd be best off avoiding it.) A beer aficionado who loves microbrews will have to search out and screen beers for problem ingredients. I have had a couple, for instance, brewed from chicory that were delicious. Of all alcoholic beverages, beer is the most hazardous, so be careful.

If you must drink beer, among the least troublesome are:

REDBRIDGE. An Anheuser Busch beer, Redbridge is brewed from sorghum (a grain), has no barley malt, and is confidently gluten-free. Carbohydrate content is a bit high at 16.4 g per bottle; drink more than one and carbohydrates begin to stack up. Bear in mind that it is brewed from sorghum and may have some issues unique to that grain.

BUD LIGHT AND MICHELOB ULTRA. Anheuser Busch's Bud Light beer is brewed from rice but also contains proteins from barley malt. The most severely gluten-sensitive should not indulge in this beer because of the potential immune cross-reactivity of barley and wheat gluten. But most of us just avoiding wheat but without gluten sensitivity can safely consume this brand without exposing ourselves to the undesirable effects of grains. Note that one 350 ml (12 fl oz) bottle of Bud Light contains 6.6 g carbohydrates. Michelob Ultra is likewise brewed from rice and barley malt, and it's low in carbohydrates with 2.6 g per 350 ml (12 fl oz) serving.

BARD'S GLUTEN-FREE BEER. Brewed from sorghum without barley malt, this beer is truly gluten-free but is still brewed from a grain. As with many of the gluten-free beers, however, it can present an excessive carbohydrate exposure if more than one is consumed (14.2 g carbohydrates per 350 ml/12 fl oz bottle). Because it is brewed from sorghum, it lacks the gliadin and gluten residues associated with wheat, rye, and barley, but contains less harmful residues of the relatively indigestible proteins of sorghum. So just beware of any undesirable reactions.

GREEN'S GLUTEN-FREE BEERS. A UK brewer, Green's provides several gluten-free choices made from sorghum, millet, buckwheat, brown rice, and "deglutenised" barley malt. They are not grain-free and so have small quantities of grain proteins. Go carefully here and make judgments based on individual experience. Carbohydrate content of these beers is slightly less than most others, ranging from 10 to 14 g per 330 ml (11 fl oz) bottle.

Spirits

Avoid vodkas brewed from wheat, which include Absolut, Grey Goose, Ketel One, SKYY, and Stolichnaya. Also avoid non-wheat but gluten-containing grain-sourced vodkas including Belvedere (rye), Finlandia (barley), and Van Gogh (wheat, barley, corn). Smirnoff is brewed from corn, which is less problematic but does have a low quantity of zein protein residues. The safest vodkas are prepared from non-grains such as grapes, potatoes, and quinoa, and are free of any grain proteins. The list of grain-free vodkas includes Chopin (potatoes) and Cîroc (grapes). Beware of flavored varieties that have been pouring into the market, as they are typically loaded with sugar or high-fructose corn syrup or both.

For those highly sensitive to grain proteins, most whiskeys are off the list since they are distilled from the mash of rye, barley, wheat, and corn. While whiskeys nearly always test below the 20 parts per million limit for gluten that the American FDA considers the safe threshold for people with celiac disease and gluten sensitivity, many of us still seem to react to them (bloating, gastrointestinal distress, joint pain). It means that many of the popular whiskeys, such as Jack Daniels (barley, rye, corn), Jameson (barley), and Bushmills (barley), carry the risk of a grain/gluten reaction. If you are among those without such extreme sensitivities, you may be fine, given the very low quantity of grain proteins.

Brandies and cognacs are generally safe since they are distilled from wines. Safe brands include Grand Marnier, Courvoisier, and Rémy Martin. There are occasional exceptions, such as Martell, that contain caramel coloring, a grain-sourced ingredient.

Rum is distilled from sugarcane and does not contain any residues of grain proteins. Look for just plain light or dark rum and avoid the flavored or spiced rums, which run the risk of a grain-based ingredient and added sugars or high-fructose corn syrup.

From a grain exposure standpoint, safe liqueurs include Kahlua (contains dairy), fruit liqueurs like triple sec and Cherry Kijafa, Amaretto di Saronno, and Bailey's Irish Cream. The most gluten-sensitive may have to avoid those blended with whiskey; while the source of whiskey is often not specified, it is typically grain. Note that liqueurs also tend to be high in sugar.

SUPPORTIVE WEB SITES
AND SOCIAL MEDIA PAGES

Official Wheat Belly Facebook page: facebook.com/ OfficialWheatBelly

The Wheat Belly Facebook page is not a place for teenage girls to giggle about boyfriends, but a place for us adults to share stories of success and hurdles to overcome, commiserate during grain withdrawal, and share or obtain advice as you proceed through your detox and onward. You are joining hundreds of thousands of other people sharing this journey with you. (It's called the "Official" Wheat Belly Facebook page because, like anything with growing worldwide popularity, there are inevitable copycats.)

Wheat Belly Recipe Central Facebook page: facebook.com/pages/ Wheat-Belly-Recipe-Central/124754534306616?ref=hl

This is the place to find or post recipes consistent with the Wheat Belly lifestyle.

The Wheat Belly Blog: wheatbellyblog.com

The Wheat Belly Blog and the Official Wheat Belly Facebook page are the two places to go for discussions and additional information about the Wheat Belly lifestyle. Updates to the program are published on the blog, as well as occasional recipes and announcements of events.

WHEAT- AND GRAIN-FREE
FOOD SOURCES

Wheat-Free Market Foods: wheatfreemarket.com

Facebook page: facebook.com/WheatFreeMarketFoods

All products made by Wheat-Free Market Foods are reviewed and approved by Dr. Davis and are therefore consistent with the Wheat Belly lifestyle. Classic Granola, Slow Toasted Flakes breakfast "cereal," Pizza Crust Mix, and other products are available online and in a growing number of grocery and health food stores. You can find nearly an entire cookbook of recipes on its Web site (under "Recipes" along the top navigation bar).

Thrive Market: thrivemarket.com

While Thrive Market, an online store for organic groceries and other products, is a paid membership site, it donates a free membership to a low-income family for every paid membership. The choices are organic, non-genetically modified, and gluten-free, and are expanding rapidly.

Radiant Life: radiantlifecatalog.com

This online retailer offers coconut oil, coconut flour, and other organic, non-genetically modified products.

nuts.com

This is an excellent online source for whole and ground nuts at reasonable prices.

PREFERRED PROBIOTIC SUPPLEMENTS

All the brands listed below meet the criteria of having high numbers of organisms in each capsule and at least a dozen (if not 30 or more) species of the varieties believed to be beneficial for bowel and overall health (based on clinical studies). Note that many mainstream brands, such as Culturelle, Align, and Activia yogurt, are not among the Wheat Belly recommended brands for various reasons, primarily for not meeting our criteria of number and diversity of microorganisms contained.

Garden of Life Ultimate Care Raw Probiotics

Renew Life Ultimate Flora Critical Care

VSL#3—Although containing only eight bacterial strains, the published track record of this preparation makes it one of our preferred probiotic sources.

COMMERCIAL SOURCES OF PREBIOTIC FIBERS/RESISTANT STARCHES

Build up your intake of these powerful prebiotic fibers gradually to minimize abdominal discomfort and bloating as you cultivate healthy bowel flora. While we aim for an intake of 20 g prebiotic fiber per day, less is needed for some of these commercial preparations. For example, no more than 5 g per day of acacia fiber and PGX achieves the desired effects (long term, though, an increase may yield greater benefits). Also, note that some of these fibers, especially PGX, are substantially water absorbent, and you will need to compensate by increasing fluid intake.

Recall that we are trying to cultivate diversity among the species composing bowel flora. You would do best by varying your prebiotic fibers several times per week.

Powders and Capsules

Inulin and fructooligosaccharides (FOS)

Purchased as powders or capsules, these fibers are closely related. Both provide a prebiotic effect to cultivate healthy species in the intestine, especially Bifidobacteria. Many preparations contain both forms.

PGX

While marketed primarily as a weight-loss supplement (by inducing satiety), this mixture of fibers also yields prebiotic effects. It is available as granules or capsules. (Avoid the Vegan Bars, as they are too high in sugars.) Start at a dose of 1.5 g twice per day and build up to 10 to 15 g per day (divided into two or three doses) over several weeks.

Prebiotin

This is a powdered form of inulin and fructooligosaccharides (FOS) and provides 4 g prebiotic fibers per teaspoon, 2 g per Stick Pac, or 4 g per Extra Strength Stick Pac (single-serve packages convenient for travel).

Renew Life Skinny Gut Organic Acacia Fiber

Provides 5 g prebiotic fibers per tablespoon.

Protein Bars

While there are more than two brands of bars on the market that contain prebiotic fibers, many also contain problem ingredients such as sugar, excessive carbohydrates, grains, or agave nectar. The bars listed below are the brands without these complicating ingredients. I find them especially useful for travel when I don't want to lug around raw potatoes or other cumbersome foods.

- Paleo Protein Bar—These low-carb bars made with egg white protein and sweetened with monk fruit contain 20 g or more isomaltooligosaccharide, a form of prebiotic fiber.

- Quest Bars—These low-carb bars provide around 17 to 18 g isomaltooligosaccharide. Choose the flavors sweetened with stevia and erythritol, rather than sucralose (which disrupts bowel flora and potentially works against the prebiotic benefits). This means choosing Banana Nut Muffin, Chocolate Peanut Butter, S'mores, Strawberry Cheesecake, Double Chocolate Chunk, Coconut Cashew, or Lemon Cream Pie.

FURTHER READING

Bowden, Jonny, and Stephen Sinatra. *The Great Cholesterol Myth: Why Lowering Your Cholesterol Won't Prevent Heart Disease—And the Statin-Free Plan That Will.* Beverly, MA: Fair Winds Press, 2012.
  If you desire further discussion on why "cholesterol testing" is a deeply flawed practice and why there are better ways to evaluate heart disease risk, Mr. Bowden and Dr. Sinatra provide a thorough and readable resource.

Davis, William. *Wheat Belly: Lose the Wheat, Lose the Weight and Find Your Path Back to Health.* London: HarperThorsons, 2014.
  This is the original book that turned the nutritional world topsy-turvy with revelations about modern wheat and its health effects.

Davis, William. *Wheat Belly Total Health: The Ultimate Grain-Free Health and Weight-Loss Life Plan.* London: Thorsons, 2015.
  The follow-up to the original book, this book details how many health conditions can be reversed with efforts that go beyond wheat elimination.

Perlmutter, David. *Brain Maker: The Power of Gut Microbes to Heal and Protect Your Brain—For Life.* New York: Little, Brown and Company, 2015.
  This is among the best resources for discussions about bowel health and bowel flora that I have come across.

Perlmutter, David. *Grain Brain: The Surprising Truth about Wheat, Carbs, and Sugar—Your Brain's Silent Killers.* New York: Little, Brown and Company, 2013.

Dr. Perlmutter's now-classic book provides extensive rationale explaining how grains and carbohydrates underlie dementia and other brain conditions.

Taubes, Gary. *Why We Get Fat and What to Do about It*. New York: Alfred A. Knopf, 2011.

Journalist Gary Taubes has proven to be one of the champions of clear thinking, thoroughly exposing the flawed science behind the cut-your-fat and cut-your-saturated-fat advice.

Teicholz, Nina. *The Big Fat Surprise: Why Butter, Meat, and Cheese Belong in a Healthy Diet*. New York: Simon and Schuster, 2014.

Nina Teicholz painstakingly dissects the bad science behind conventional advice to curtail fat to reduce heart disease risk.

Grain-Free Cookbooks

Davis, William. *Wheat Belly Cookbook: 150 Delicious Wheat-Free Recipes for Effortless Weight Loss & Optimum Health*. London: Thorsons, 2015.

Davis, William. *Wheat Belly 30-Minute (or Less!) Cookbook: 200 Quick and Simple Wheat-Free and Grain-Free Recipes*. London: Thorsons, 2015.

Emmerich, Maria. *The Art of Healthy Eating—Savory: Grain Free Low Carb Reinvented*. Amazon Digital Services, 2012.

Mason, Hayley, and Bill Staley. *Gather: The Art of Paleo Entertaining*. Las Vegas: Victory Belt Publishing, 2013.

Walker, Danielle. *Against All Grain: Delectable Paleo Recipes to Eat Well & Feel Great*. Las Vegas: Victory Belt Publishing, 2013.

GENERAL INDEX

Underscored page references indicate sidebars.

RECIPE INDEX